DEDICATION

I would like to dedicate this work to my husband, Rick, and to the rest of my family. Thank you for the love and unwavering support.

Kathleen L. Sitzman

This book is dedicated to those closest to me, my family.

My earliest memory is of my mom and dad bringing home my baby sister. Little did I know it was the luckiest day of my life. Thanks, Karen, for being my best friend through life. You know more secrets about me than anyone else alive or dead.

To my husband, John, thanks for loving me, sharing me with nursing, and being my "biggest fan"!

And to my children, of whom I am so proud. To Matthew, who fights everyday to protect the rights of those without a voice; Elizabeth, who runs her own business and is the best little mother I have ever seen; and to Tera, who is just beginning to find out who she will be in this world. Whatever she chooses, I know her love of others and caring spirit will bring much joy to the lives she touches.

Thanks to you all for loving me, believing in me, and making life so precious and sweet.

Lisa Wright Eichelberger

Contents

PART V

THEORIES THAT DEFY CLASSIFICATION 173

PART VI

CONCLUSION 203

New Companion Web Site for
Understanding the Work of Nurse Theorists: A Creative Beginning

http://nursing.jbpub.com

The newly revised companion Web site for this book contains numerous learning and studying resources for students and a variety of tools for instructors.

Feel free to use any of the resources at this companion Web site to help you study and to better understand nursing theory and the theorists discussed in the book.

Select features of the companion Web site include:

For Students:

- Interactive glossary
- Crossword puzzles
- Quizzes
- Web links

For Instructors:

- PowerPoint slides
- TestBank
- Teaching strategies
- Discussion questions with suggested answers
- Theory art gallery

FOREWORD

This work in nursing theory opens new doors and opens up new horizons of learning, studying, embodying, and using nursing theory. It is an introduction to creative scholarship, inviting new, engaging, artistic, aesthetic, imaginary, and evocative approaches to entering into, and participating in, inspirited and inspired learning. *Understanding the Work of Nurse Theorists: A Creative Beginning* takes us into new territory for teaching and learning theory, while interacting with the depth of philosophical, idealistic, ethical, theoretical constructs, concepts, and meanings embedded in diverse theories. This unique and original approach to nursing theory is not otherwise offered when considering learning and teaching *nursing theory*.

Sitzman and Eichelberger have a special grasp and postmodern view of the significance and insights that can be gained from diverse approaches to learning that draw upon all ways of knowing, being, and learning. They offer an original pedagogical perspective that integrates art and artistry with concepts and methods of thinking while probing philosophical insights through concrete, original, creative-artistic learning experiences and exercises that bring theory to life and make it a living process. By doing so, the reader/students are co-creating the learning–discovery process.

This text opens the hearts and minds of the readers and students to let in fresh air and present new ways of learning. The text of theory is to be read as an open, evolving text, rather than a closed, set, stable subject.

This text takes us into the heart of the theorists' thinking, while assisting the student with self-created challenges to use creativity, curiosity, thoughtfulness, and joy of discovery. The authors help to illuminate new depths of learning for seeing the relevance and dynamic living nature of theory-in-action in our personal/professional lives and work. It is a book that takes us into the new world of learning and teaching, beyond the sterile rote, staid thinking that often dominates our views of theory.

It is through works such as this that nurses will learn that they are the theories; theories are not separate and detached from their being, but a living thought system that both informs and guides nursing into this new century, while sustaining the finest of the historical heritage and roots of nursing. *Understanding the Work of Nurse Theorists: A Creative Beginning* is a book for beginners and experts alike, inspiriting and inspiring a new generation of students, nurses, theorists, and theories.

Jean Watson, PhD, RN, HNC, FAAN
Distinguished Professor of Nursing
Murchinson-Scoville Chair of Caring Science
University of Colorado Health Sciences Center

PREFACE

Nursing theories are the creative products of nurses who seek to thoughtfully describe relationships and interactions that exist within nursing practice. Theories address the many questions that confront nurses daily. Theories are multilayered and consist of numerous tangible and intangible components. Attempts at initial understanding of complex nursing theories are often overwhelming and intensely unsatisfying for beginning students.

Most undergraduate nursing students are exposed to nursing theory in a limited way during the process of completing basic nursing education. Unfortunately, the attitude of students taking nursing theory for the first time is often one of dread. Many express the opinion that theory has little relevance for present or future clinical practice. Often, it becomes the task of nursing educators to try and convey the idea that theory is important for the continued growth and development of nursing practice. This text is designed for first-time nursing theory students who may believe that theory will be irrelevant, uninspiring, and difficult to grasp.

When beginning the study of nursing theory, two things must be made clear to students:

1. Nursing theory is relevant to present and future practice.
2. Students are not expected to become nurse theorists or experts.

Traditional theory teaching methods have not always been effective in communicating the above two points to students. In theory classes, papers and other writing-based projects often are assigned in which the student is required to somehow comprehend the complex web of ideas that constitutes nursing theory and then expound on how theory informs practice or applies to personal professional experience. Producing coherent assignments about nursing theory requires a relatively advanced level of understanding that may not be accessible to students with limited exposure to the material. Students expend a great deal of energy in the struggle to produce "perfect" assignments with acceptable levels of understanding, and in the course of this struggle, teaching/learning opportunities to draw the student in, to experience the Gestalt and beauty of nursing theory, melt away. After struggling through what often seems to be an exercise in confusion and futility, many students vow never to study nursing theory again after formal education is complete.

Most currently available theory texts are more complex and detailed than what is needed, or desired, for classes taught at the beginning level, and therefore may be more confusing than helpful for most students. Unfortunately, this often leads to either frustrated students and instructors, or (in response to the frustration), the elimination of all but cursory content at the baccalaureate level. If students are instead encouraged to approach the challenge of comprehending nursing theory from the position of a beginner's mind, with creativity, curiosity, thoughtfulness, and joy, then the learning process has the power to clarify and illuminate depths of nursing theory in ways that will hold meaning for the student long after the class is over.

This text offers a different approach to teaching and learning nursing theory. The essential definitions and basic concepts are presented along with a brief overview of the most common nursing theories. However, what is unique about this text is the use of art to illuminate nursing theories. This method mobilizes creativity for the construction of personal meaning. In encouraging creativity through the use of the universal language of art, students become engaged and active learners. When this text and learning activities are used as a guide for learning, students do not sit passively in a classroom, memorizing definitions and facts. The activities outlined in this text are visual, tactile, and kinesthetic. Students are able to read, see, touch, and manipulate the learning materials. Although comprehensive understanding of theory (perfect understanding) is not the intent or result of this creative approach, a light of beginning understanding will be ignited by this approach.

A quote by Leonard Cohen says it well:

Ring the bells that still can ring,
forget your perfect offering.
There is a crack in everything.
That's how the light gets in (Schiller, 1994, p. 26).

Another way to explain this creative approach is the chocolate chip cookie example. As with nursing theory, a chocolate chip cookie consists of numerous components, both tangible (i.e., color, texture, size) and intangible (i.e., how tempting it may look to the casual passerby). To convey a complete understanding of all that is a chocolate chip cookie, a teacher might thoroughly describe, diagram, and explain down to the chemical and atomic levels exactly what one is. The information obtained during this type of teaching/learning exchange would be undoubtedly accurate in every detail. Unfortunately, if the student has never tasted a chocolate chip cookie, the prospect of trying to appreciate and understand one seems, at best, bewildering, and, at worst, frustrating busywork. And so it is with the introductory study of nursing theory.

The alternative learning methods suggested in this handbook offer beginning opportunities for learning through visual and experiential pathways, similar to tasting a cookie before studying it in-depth. The methods are also meant to support personal discovery and the construction of individual meaning, for instance, "This cookie tastes pretty interesting! I want to learn more!" This is a somewhat back-door approach to generating learning moments by offering glimpses of the complete picture before attempting to dissect and understand the complexity of the components. Most nursing theories are unquestionably complex, however, simplicity of explanation is used in this text in order to foster freedom of thought and creativity and to draw the student in so that in-depth study will be more willingly embraced later.

Companion Web Site: *http://nursing.jbpub.com*

Students and instructors: Don't forget to visit the complete companion Web site that accompanies this book!

- **Students** will find various tools to help them study, from an interactive glossary to quick quizzes!

- **Instructors** will find resources to help facilitate classroom discussions and direct their lectures!

Introduction to Theory in Nursing

What Is Nursing Theory?

Nursing theories are the creative products of nurses who seek (or sought) to thoughtfully describe the many aspects of nursing in ways that could be studied, evaluated, and used by other nurses. In other words, theory is an attempt to explain patterns and relationships found in nursing phenomena. Nurse theorists are people who are or have been nurses, have thought deeply about how one might describe the phenomenon of nursing, and then tried in their own way, from their own perspective, to record their thoughts and observations based on professional and personal experiences. Each theory is as unique as the individual(s) who created it.

In many cases, the creators of nursing theories did not set out to "become" nurse theorists. For the most part, theories evolved, and continue to evolve, out of creative attempts to describe nursing phenomenon in ways that made sense to the theorists and others. Published nursing theories stimulate formal debate, exploration, and research regarding the nature and process of nursing. Theories give nurses different ways of viewing reality, such as expanding awareness of concepts never before considered, organizing care activities, and providing opportunities for reflection and the formation of opinions. Nursing theories are formal tools for communication that enable experienced nurses to communicate specific perceptions about nursing in a structured way so that others have an opportunity to study, evaluate, participate in, and add to an ongoing dialogue meant to address questions such as:

- What do nurses do?
- What makes nursing unique from other healthcare-related professions?
- What is wholistic nursing care?
- What is meant by terms such as "wellness" and "illness"?
- Do certain nursing actions measurably improve client outcomes?
- What differentiates excellent nursing care from marginal nursing care?
- Is nursing a job, a vocation, a profession, or a combination of all three?
- Is the core of nursing "caring" or technical skill mastery?
- Is nursing meant to be an independent profession or an auxiliary component of the medical profession?
- Should nursing practice formally encompass the metaphysical? Spiritual?
- How should phenomena that cannot be concretely measured through the five senses be addressed in nursing?

These are only a few of a myriad of questions and concerns addressed by nursing theories. The focus of a particular theory depends on the concurrent historical/political/social/professional environment and the personal and professional experiences of the theorist. Because there are wide-ranging issues associated with nursing practice, theories may be created to address broad or very narrow aspects of the profession.

For the purposes of organization and ease of understanding, nursing theories can be placed into three loosely defined categories:

1. Definitions of nursing in general (philosophies)
2. Discussions of broad nursing practice areas (grand theories)
3. Assertions about specific nursing actions, processes, or concepts (middle-range theories)

Some nursing theories may fit into more than one category, depending on how they are interpreted and used by individuals. There is no firm rule regarding what category a specific theory fits into. In fact, there is much debate surrounding theory development and evaluation. The questions and ambiguity surrounding these ongoing debates may be disconcerting to those new to the study of theory because there never seems to be a *correct* answer or viewpoint. The first assignment in any study of nursing theory should be to become comfortable with ambiguity. For example, there are ongoing debates over categorical determinations or differences in terms, such as *theory* versus *model* versus *theoretical framework*. There will probably never be a final resolution to these debates because of the great variety of viewpoints among nursing scholars, only continued professional dialogues that stimulate exploration and learning. Because ambiguity is quite often a feature of the study of nursing theory, productive learning approaches include listening, evaluating, reading, adopting another's position to assess personal fit, formulating an informed opinion, and realizing that firm answers do not always apply.

Informed opinion based on scholarly study *is* a valid approach in deciding what category a theory might fit into at any given time. A scholar, whether beginning or expert, is expected to have an opinion based on logical, rational thought that can be explained. Making informed judgments about theories may seem a daunting task for a beginner; methods for making such determinations will be discussed in Chapter 5. More complete discussions and examples of theory categories are contained in Parts II, III, and IV. Be aware that this text is just one approach for "making sense" of nursing theories. Use the broad categories and definitions presented here or other classification systems with the awareness that there will be variations and debates within the literature regarding nursing theory. Continued debates, however, do not diminish the importance of nursing theory for the profession. As a matter of fact, nursing theory and its role in nursing research has done more to advance the scholarship of nursing over the last 40 years than any other nursing endeavor. Nursing theory has served as a framework for inquiry that has allowed the profession to create its own body of knowledge. For now, it may be helpful to remember that theories, though to some extent abstract and ambiguous, exist to help nurses explain and guide the very real practice world around them.

Why Are Theories Important in Nursing?

Theories provide structure and order for guiding and improving professional practice, teaching and learning activities, and research. Exactly how might a theory be important for everyday nursing activities? Surely theories are too far removed from "nurses in the trenches" to really impact much of anything, right? This may not be necessarily so, as demonstrated by the examples in this chapter.

The following is an example of a theory influencing professional practice.

Assume a practicing nurse learns about a nursing theory that describes the "whole" of nursing practice as consisting of activities in technical, ethical, and wholistic care areas. Before learning about this theory, the nurse had focused the bulk of his/her professional effort on mastering technical skills. After learning about this theory, the nurse actively explores ethical and wholistic care concerns by reading articles about these topics in two professional journals that are delivered monthly to his/her home and by searching for related information on the Internet. The inclusion of ethical and wholistic principles into professional practice enriches personal job satisfaction and effectiveness. Client satisfaction also improves. The nurse shares information about this theory and how it has the potential to enrich professional practice with a few colleagues. Pretty soon, the nursing staff on the medical unit where the nurse works decides to adopt the theory as a formal guide for unitwide practice. It will also be shared during orientation of new nursing staff and will be used as a guide when decisions are made regarding unit practices and policies.

The following is an example of how theories might influence teaching and learning activities.

A small university is constructing a nursing program that will provide an RN to BSN degree in nursing to qualified students who complete the program of study. There are numerous ways of teaching nursing, and there are thousands of textbooks, computer programs, and study formats to consider when constructing a program. What classes will be offered and in what order? What is the most important, central concept that all students should come away with when the course of study is completed? In order to clarify what direction to take in developing this program, educators will need to first decide what theories will guide educational practices. Most nursing programs in the United States base programs on one or more nursing theories, in addition to basic educational theories. In the case of this small university, it is decided to base the curriculum on three theories: two broad nursing theories that identify "wholistic caring" as the central concept in nursing practice and one other, more specific, theory that describes a sequential process by which nurses may effectively provide "hands-on" client care. After selecting these theories as a guide, it then becomes possible to consciously create a course of study focused on the principles of "caring" put forth in the first two selected theories, with the third, more specific theory providing a framework for selecting and sequencing course material.

The following is an example of how a theory might guide a research activity.

Theories often provide the basis for the creation of questions that will be asked during research activities. Theories may also clarify ways in which to *focus* observations and data collection. For example, Jordan, a nurse in the newborn intensive care unit (NICU), wishes to learn if mothers who are allowed unlimited visiting time with their infants experience more effective mother–infant bonding than mothers who are asked to adhere to a restricted visiting schedule. Jordan discovers that there are several nursing journal articles about mother–infant bonding research studies, and as a result of these past studies, theories have been created to describe the process of successful mother–infant bonding. Jordan finds one theory that makes the most sense in terms of personal professional experience and uses it as a guide in creating her study. The theory Jordan selects describes an eight-step process of bonding that starts with the mother's realization of pregnancy and culminates in successful postpartum bonding between mother and infant. Jordan decides to observe for the presence of these eight steps when assessing the progress of bonding in both groups of mothers and infants (unrestricted vs. restricted visiting). During the course of the study, Jordan may find that the eight steps described in the previous study accurately describe what is observed (validating the theory) or the eight steps may not apply at all to what is observed (not supporting the theory). In either instance, Jordan will be performing two vital functions associated with nursing research: gathering data that may be helpful in clarifying mother–infant bonding for NICU clients and assessing the validity and applicability of a previously created nursing theory. If Jordan's study validates the eight-step process, this might provide support for use of this theory for the development of programs that will support optimal mother–infant bonding in multiple NICU settings. If Jordan's study does not support the eight-step process, then valuable information regarding directions for future studies will be provided.

In a general sense, theory development supports independence of the nursing profession by creating forums where nurses have opportunities to develop and support unique professional visions. Theories specific to nursing help differentiate nursing from other care-related professions. Because nursing encompasses a variety of professional activities, there is room for a corresponding variety of nursing theories, all meant to accurately describe nursing in one way or another.

A logical question at this point might be, "Is it possible to firmly determine which theories are *correct*?" Because scholarly, well-educated nurses have created these theories, does it mean that others must accept them as truth? Just because there is a significant body of research and publications using a particular nursing theory in practice does not mean that this theory is right for every nurse.

Likewise, there is no single theory, or group of theories, that is more correct than another. Nursing practice is inexorably tied to human interactions and experiences; precise and unwavering conclusions are often not possible.

It is up to the individual to determine if a particular theory makes sense after evaluation and comparison with personal values and belief systems and if it adds value to education, practice, and research. In other words, it is the responsibility of each nurse to independently evaluate if a given theory resonates with personal professional practice. What feels "correct" for one nurse may not necessarily feel "correct" for another nurse.

Also, nurses and nursing theories are dynamic, shifting, growing entities, therefore, a theory that did not initially seem important to an individual nurse may become more important as the nurse matures or as the theory evolves through time. Usefulness of a particular theory is strongly related to personal and professional relevance at any given point in time.

Please be aware that it takes courage and vision to present to the world beliefs (theories) based on professional observations. Even if you do not agree with or appreciate a particular theory, please respect the intellect, introspection, and tremendous amount of work it took for the theorist to create a formal presentation of ideas for you to evaluate. Each model or theory is a representation of creativity and diversity within nursing ranks. In diversity there can be strength if we allow ourselves to celebrate the unique (and equally valid) visions of our colleagues that make up the totality of nursing.

The Development of Nursing Theories

The Nurse Theorists

As stated in Chapter 1, most nurse theorists did not set out to create a nursing theory. Most began constructing a theory as a way to improve the care delivered to clients, whether through direct clinical practice or through the education of nurses. The theorists were risk takers with lifelong commitments to the nursing profession. They viewed nursing as a career rather than as an alternative to marriage, which was the view of many nurses during the 1940s, 1950s, and 1960s. These theorists had broad, well-rounded educational backgrounds and a variety of interests. They were inquisitive, bold, and unafraid to question or challenge the status quo. The demands of their professional lives were great, and their home lives suffered, causing one nursing leader to remark that the early great leaders needed a "wife" to assist them or manage the personal dimension of their lives (R. Schlotfeldt, personal communication with Lisa Eichelberger, 1982). Most of the early theorists made professional choices that affected their personal lives, and most never married or had children. Interestingly, two major universities were responsible for educating most of the early nurse theorists: Peplau, Henderson, Hall, Abdellah, Orlando, Wiedenbach, King, and Rogers all graduated from either Columbia University's Teachers College in New York or Yale University in New Haven, Connecticut.

Why Theories Were Developed

Theory development was an integral part of modern nursing, as evidenced by Nightingale's *Notes on Nursing: What It Is and What It Is Not*, published in 1859. This small book was the first of its kind to theoretically describe the nature of nursing. Research was also an integral part of modern nursing, as evidenced by Nightingale's extensive research projects and publications related to examining the economics and efficacy of army hospitals. Unfortunately, Nightingale's examples of theory development and research were not carried forth. It would be nearly 100 years before nursing theory and research were again considered essential for nurses.

It was not until the 1950s that nurse scholars started to develop *nursing* theories. This occurred during a time when professional thought in nursing was moving toward conceptualizing nursing as a profession based on science rather than as a trade-based apprenticeship. Also at this time, nursing education was in transition, with the education and training of nurses moving into college-level educational institutions and out of hospital-based training schools (Kalisch & Kalisch, 1995).

In the 1960s, the first doctoral programs in nursing were established (Chinn & Kramer, 1999). Prior to the 1960s most nurses who wished to pursue a doctorate, did so in related fields such as sociology, education, psychology, and anthropology and then adapted theories from those fields for use in nursing. This approach was initially helpful; however, it became apparent that nursing was unique and contained many aspects not addressed in theories from other disciplines. Other disciplines from which nursing theories were adapted were not immersed in the *actual, real-life particulars* of embodiment; that is, professionally managing the specifics of humans in various states of wellness. For instance, nurses often assess a client's mental, social, and spiritual well-being while at the same time giving a bed bath, evaluating skin integrity, assessing the stage of healing of a surgical wound, and observing for patency of a urinary bladder catheter. Psychologists, sociologists, and anthropologists would generally *not* be expected to provide intimate physical assessment and care while evaluating the psychological and social concerns of an individual or group of individuals. Because of this difference, theories from other related disciplines were (and are) applicable to nursing only in a limited sense. Nursing leaders began to understand that if nursing was to develop its own body of knowledge, the creation of *nursing* theory was essential, and doctoral level *nursing* education and research were critical (Wilde, 1999).

Why the Theorists Created Theories

When the biographies and works of the individual theorists are examined, it becomes apparent that the impetus for developing a theory, model, or framework was for two primary reasons: to further nursing as a scholarly profession and to organize and improve the delivery of nursing care. Almost without exception, the nurse theorists created their theories, at least in part, as a result of their direct experiences in practice and their desire to improve practice, whether clinical or classroom based. Imogene King (General Systems Framework) and Martha Rogers (Science of Unitary Human Beings) stated specifically that they developed a conceptual framework/theory because of their concern over the lack of nursing knowledge. These two theorists felt that this knowledge was essential to the development of nursing as a science. Other reasons for theory development given by early theorists were that theories could be tools to provide structure for the improvement of clinical practice, teaching nursing students effectively, or organizing a nursing curriculum.

How Theorists Created Theories

The development of nursing theory started with Nightingale and her astute and mindful observations of actual nursing practice environments. The idea that nursing theory comes from practice is consistent with Dickoff and James's classic theory development article (1968) that says theory about a practice discipline must come from actual practice experience. Discovery of knowledge, concepts, and relationships among and between concepts about the discipline occur when practitioners are immersed in practice. It is through reflective thinking that practitioners are able to gain insight into the patterns that may exist in the practice arena (Johns, 1995).

Creating a theory is like constructing a complex puzzle (Van Sell & Kalofissudis, 2003). The nurse theorists relate very similar stories as to how they approached theory development. They reflected upon personal and professional experiences to make sense of worldviews and then put together the pieces of the puzzle with the goal of coherent description and explanation.

The nurse theorists used reflection to gain understanding and to glean new knowledge from practice experience. Reflection is an intentional undertaking that requires time and commitment. The purpose of reflection is to allow practitioners to examine clinical anecdotes and resolve contradictions between what the nurse desires to achieve and what is experienced in actual practice, with the goal to achieve more effective outcomes (Johns, 1993). Reflection was described by many of the nurse theorists as one way to generate nursing theory. However, frustration, confusion, the need for organization of content, and the need for a way to communicate outcomes to others also proved helpful in stimulating theory development (Helene Fuld Video Series, 1987–1988,1989).

Theorists wanted to improve the nursing profession and also improve daily clinical nursing care. Reflective practice allowed them to learn and draw conclusions through lived experiences. Nurse theorists sought ways to represent the realities and relationships found within nursing practice. Theories were developed to enhance practice either directly, by stimulating practice-based thinking through reflection, or indirectly, through further development of theory (Ingram, 1991). Said another way, the theorists observed a phenomenon in practice, reflected on it over time, compared it to what was known, and determined goodness of fit and usefulness. Then the phenomenon was named, classified, and categorized, and relationships/interrelationships were described (Peden, 1998).

An example of practice-based theory development can be found in the work of Peplau and her use of participant observation with depressed women (Peplau, 1989). Peplau's work was the earliest published work (1969) after Nightingale. Peplau used several methods of observation, such as interviews, spectator observation, and random observation. She recorded her observations of the nurses and patients, classified and categorized the data, assigned meaning at different levels of abstraction within the phenomenon, and, finally, interpreted the observations in the context of the phenomena. Patterns emerged throughout this process, and Peplau was able to develop interventions from the patterns that helped the patient gain interpersonal competencies during illness (Peden, 1998). It was through this process that Peplau developed her model of Interpersonal Relations in Nursing.

Testing of Theory

Theory, practice and research are interrelated and interdependent. Theory, once conceptualized, must be tested. While theories were being developed in the 1950s and 1960s, doctoral programs in nursing were being established and masters programs were becoming entrenched. Research programs were established, and nurses began to conduct nursing research. Columbia University's Teachers College primarily used a biomedical model for its research focus in the 1950s and concentrated on the roles of nurses. In the 1960s, Yale School of Nursing's research focus was on nursing as a process (George, 2002).

During the subsequent decades, the number and quality of nursing research efforts grew significantly in number, and the emergence of nursing as a science began. However, there was debate over the methodology being used to study nursing concepts. Since the 1920s, the academic community primarily used the scientific method of discovery, also known as Logical Positivism, which is based on the assumption that objective truth could be discovered through rigorous observation and experimentation. According to Logical Positivism, a statement or theory is meaningful and adds to knowledge through objective verification: measuring, observing, and quantifying for the purpose of generalizing (Ayers, 1990).

During the late 20th century, much debate occurred between the social, philosophical, educational, spiritual, and scientific disciplines, and many academic scholars started to view science, theory building, and the generation of knowledge as more of a process rather than as a way to create a "solution" or "discover the truth." The idea of flexibility with regards to the generation of knowledge and theory development started gaining acceptance, and the process of theory development in more recent times has begun to encompass phenomena that cannot be concretely measured and quantified using methods based on the tenets of Logical Positivism (Allmark, 2003). Given the fact that nursing deals with human beings and controlled experimentation is very often impossible, many nurse researchers use qualitative research methods. These qualitative methods, along with alternative approaches, often referred to as "postmodern" methods (Crotty, 1998) are sometimes not fully embraced in the scientific community. Some nurses find these postmodern approaches liberating, others (who still accept Logical Positivism and scientific method as the "gold standard" for knowledge development) are skeptical of these new approaches.

It is normal for individuals to develop opinions that favor one method of theory development and inquiry over another. The kind or type of research one chooses should be dependent on the questions to be answered, rather than on the method of inquiry deemed "acceptable" in most academic circles. Some important questions associated with nursing phenomena that cannot be answered using a controlled, experimental approach lend themselves well to exploration through postmodern methods. An example of such a question might be, "What is the experience of parenting a chronically ill child?" Other important nursing questions can be answered only through strict scientific methods of inquiry. An example of this type of question might be "Do axillary temperature measurements in newborns accurately reflect core body temperature?" Approaches spanning Logical Positivism to postmodern methods are essential because of the need for varied tools to use in describing the manifold aspects of nursing practice. All methods contribute to the development of nursing knowledge.

Evaluating a Theory

When evaluating a theory, it is helpful to use a stepwise process, understanding that nursing theories have common components that should be present in some form for others to understand and appreciate the information conveyed. The first step when trying to understand and evaluate a theory is to identify the presence (or absence) of the following six components (Tomey & Alligood, 2002):

1. What concepts are presented that list and classify the nursing components of interest?
2. How does the theory define person, health, environment, and nursing?
3. What are the specific statements that clarify exactly what the theory is trying to describe?
4. What types of definitions are used in the theory?
   a. *Theoretical definitions* explain the nature of something in a broad sense and may not be immediately applicable to everyday activities.
   b. *Operational definitions* are meant to explain exactly how something works (e.g., Exactly what is meant by "wellness"? What are the observable or measurable signs that a person is experiencing a high degree of wellness?)

5. What are the links or relationships between terms, concepts, and theoretical assertions?

6. How are the concepts and statements organized? (Simple to complex? Linear? Highly structured? Unstructured?)

After forming a basic understanding of what the selected theory is about and identifying the presence or absence of the six components, it is time to evaluate the theory in terms of personal and professional relevance. Consider the following questions based on information found in Chinn and Kramer (1999):

1. What is your gut response to the basic tenets put forth in this theory? Does it make sense in relation to your own professional experience?

2. How clear is this theory? Can you "buy into it"? What factors made this theory either clear or unclear to you? (e.g., a feeling or belief that you have held or specificity to a clinical area that you are either familiar or unfamiliar with.)

3. How simple is it? Could you easily describe the overall ideas presented in the theory to a colleague?

4. How general is this theory? Could it be used in many types of nursing settings or is it limited to a selected type of nursing–client situation?

5. How much research exists in current literature that uses this theory as its framework or theoretical base? Choose a time frame (e.g., the years between 1999 and 2003) and conduct a literature search. Is the amount of research using this theory increasing, decreasing, or staying the same?

6. Evaluate the potential impact this theory would most likely have on your current nursing practice. If you used this theory, how significantly would it impact your practice?

Use these steps to gain a basic understanding of each theory presented in this handbook, as well as other theories of interest. The point of studying and evaluating a theory is to systematically identify meaningful components, evaluate personal relevance, and then apply new knowledge or understandings where applicable. Continued study and evaluation supports the formation of meaningful insights and opinions that will ultimately deepen professional practice. The most important questions to ask when evaluating theories are:

- Does it resonate with long-held professional insights?
- Does it stimulate new ways of thinking?
- Does it provide fresh viewpoints?

If the answer to any of these questions is "yes," then the theory warrants further exploration.

Theories That Define Nursing or Discuss Nursing in a General Sense: Philosophies

Using the Art
of Georges Seurat
to Envision Philosophies

The work of some nurse theorists may be classified as *philosophies*. Nursing theories that are classified as philosophies in this text are those created by Nightingale, Henderson, Wiedenbach, and Watson. Philosophies about *nursing in general* seek to define and document what nursing *is*. A *philosophy* is a system of beliefs regarding the general nature of all things, particularly morality, ethics, and how the world should be viewed. Nursing philosophies address the question, "How does nursing fit into the universe?" Nursing practice consists of many realms of activity, so philosophies of *nursing in general* have multiple components that are meant to categorize and clarify the scope and depth of professional activities on a personal and also a global level. The term *professional activities* may include tasks and technical skills, moral/ethical behaviors, personal growth and development, personal knowledge, and professional aesthetic expression (Chinn & Kramer, 1999). Philosophies, therefore, are broad and multidimensional, encompassing both science and art.

Envision the paintings of postimpressionist painter Georges Seurat (1859–1891) when exploring theories that seek to define nursing in general. Seurat perfected a painting technique called pointillism to create vibrant depictions of everyday life in 19th-century France. Pointillism is a technique in which tiny points, or dots, of pure color are painstakingly applied to a canvas. The human eye actively "mixes" the colors when viewing the work from a distance of a few feet away or more, thus creating innumerable shades, hues, and depths in the mind's eye. When viewed up close, it is clear that Seurat's works are made up of individual dots, or points, of color. There is beauty in the close-up view because of the brilliance and contrast of each individual dot in relation to the other dots. The play of light on the dots creates the effect of many different shades (see Color Plate 5.1 in the color insert).

Perceptions of Seurat's work vary widely among individual viewers and are unique to each person because each "mind's eye" processes the visual input a little differently, especially from a close-up view when only dots of color are perceived. Commonalities of perception become most evident when Seurat's paintings are viewed from far away, when the dots merge into a colorful picture of people, places, and activities. When viewed from a distance, most observers agree that the painting entitled A *Sunday on La Grande Jatte* depicts people out for a stroll in the park (see Color Plate 5.2 in the color insert).

In Seurat's works, there is unity and form, and at the same time, a subtle awareness of the interplay between the individual points of color and the larger composition. The color tones may evoke happy, sad, festive, calm, pensive, or other moods. *Bathers at Asnières*, created by Seurat in 1884, evokes calmness and a feeling of contented leisure. The brightness and use of color convey afternoon warmth (see Color Plate 5.3 in the color insert).

Seurat's paintings are finite works, with specific themes and bounded visual representations. However, the many points of color within each work seem to merge with the light and color in the surrounding environment to create a feeling of boundlessness.

Theories that explore or describe the phenomenon of nursing in general are similar to Seurat's paintings because each theory is made of distinct points meant to be mixed by the mind's eye so that an impression of nursing as a whole may be formed by the viewer. Most nurses are able to agree on the general concepts presented in theories or descriptions regarding nursing in general, much like those who agree that A *Sunday on La Grande Jatte* depicts people out for a Sunday stroll at the park.

When assessing the many discreet components that make up a general nursing theory or description, individual nurses may have very different impressions about specific meanings because of the unique ways in which the mind processes bits of information, much like differing perceptions of up-close viewers of Seurat's works, wherein the dots of color are processed differently by each person's "mind's eye." Often, disagreements among nurses regarding the content or applicability of a general theory arise from the "close-up" rather than the "far away" view.

Theories meant to describe or define nursing in a general sense also convey boundlessness, much like the boundlessness evident in Seurat's paintings, in which the light and color in the painting seem to merge with light and color outside the bounds of the canvas. Similarly, in studying general or descriptive theories, one tends to merge personal nursing experiences into the structure of the theory in an attempt to find resonance and meaning, thereby expanding the bounds of the theory into real-life practice. When reading about theories meant to describe nursing in a general sense, assess the information contained in each theory or description from two different vantage points:

- Close-up: What dots of color (ideas) are contained in this theory or description? List the individual ideas (dots of color) that make up the complete picture.
- From a distance: What is the overall composition of this work? What is the "picture", or central idea, that best exemplifies the theory in general? Describe, draw, or obtain a visual representation of it.

Learning Activities

Follow steps one through six to create your own visual images using pointillism (use Color Plate 5.1 in the color insert as a guide):

1. Gather painting supplies, including watercolor or cardstock-weight paper, acrylic or watercolor paints, and cotton-tipped swabs.
2. Using a pencil, lightly outline simple shapes or other forms on the paper.
3. Using cotton-tipped swabs, dab different colors of paint within and around the shapes previously outlined. Fill each shape with two or three different colors of dots.

4. Experiment with different colors by choosing one or two colors that will appear, or repeat, throughout the picture. Dab several dots of unique color along with several dots of your chosen repeating color(s) inside the drawn shapes until each shape is filled with colors. Keep dabbing until all of the different shapes (and most of the other spaces on the paper) are filled with color.

5. Look at the finished work close up. Notice how easy it is to differentiate the various dots of color and how challenging it is to discern those basic shapes that were drawn on the paper earlier and each filled with specific combinations of colors.

6. Now look at the finished work from at least 30 feet away. Notice how it becomes difficult to distinguish individual colors and it becomes easier to distinguish those larger basic shapes that were penciled in at the beginning and then filled with specific combinations of colors. (Nursing philosophies are a lot like this; under close scrutiny, they tend to look like a composition made up of unrelated points with little rhyme or reason; however, when viewed more generally, or from far away, it is easier to discern the gist of the philosophy.)

7. Go to the Jones and Bartlett Web site for this text at *http://nursing.jbpub.com* and explore the Web links listed for this chapter.

Feel free to use these blank pages as a canvas for your learning activities.

Florence Nightingale's Definition of Nursing

Florence Nightingale (1820–1910) was the second daughter of a wealthy, well-educated, aristocratic English family. Nightingale lived during the Victorian era, an era when upper- and middle-class women were expected to either marry a well-off gentleman or remain with relatives and tend to social and household duties. Nightingale's father highly valued education and provided Nightingale with rigorous tutoring in mathematics, languages, religion, and philosophy. She was a gifted learner and found pleasure and fulfillment in her studies.

Much to the dismay of her family, Nightingale decided that a life of service to mankind was preferable to traditional Victorian marriage or spinsterhood. She completed 3 months of formal nurse training at a Protestant hospital in Germany and then returned to England where she started inspecting and writing about conditions in hospitals, reformatories, and charitable institutions. In 1853, Nightingale became the superintendent of the Hospital for Invalid Gentlewomen in London. In 1854, Nightingale took 38 marginally trained nurses to Scutari, Turkey, during the Crimean War to minister to between 3000 and 4000 injured and dying British soldiers wounded in battle. When she first arrived in Scutari, the mortality rate for those admitted to the crude army hospital was 60% because of filthy conditions, poor nutrition, and utter despair.

When Nightingale returned to England, the mortality rate stood at just over 1% because Nightingale and her nurses dramatically improved hygiene, nutrition, and the level of care to the patients at Scutari. Nightingale became a celebrity in England because of her highly successful efforts in the Crimean War. After returning from the Crimea, Nightingale opened nurse training schools and worked toward the reform of army hospitals. Nightingale used the mathematical skills taught to her by her father to produce statistical analyses of cost and mortality rates associated with running military hospitals.

Through prolific writings, Nightingale expressed the vision that nursing was a vocation and a noble undertaking that required discipline and training. In 1859, Nightingale wrote a slim volume entitled *Notes on Nursing: What It Is and What It Is Not*. In this book, Nightingale expressed the belief that all women at some time or another would be called upon to "nurse" family or friends, and though "nurses" themselves may or may not have been formally trained, the act of *nursing* required educated and meticulous planning by those wishing to provide effective nursing care (Nightingale, 1859). Nightingale's slim volume, prolific personal and published writings, as well as the establishment of Nightingale nurse training schools, influenced the development of nursing from the Victorian era and into the present time (Kalisch & Kalisch, 1995).

During her lifetime of service and prolific writing, Nightingale did not specifically set out to create a nursing "theory"; however, she did endeavor to define what nursing *was*. Nightingale discussed many broad moral, spiritual, and personal aspects of what a nurse "should be" in her extant writings, and this is why her published opinions about nursing fall roughly into the category of a philosophy. Recalling the pointillism exhibited in Seurat's paintings, the different points of color (or palette) that might make up Nightingale's rendering of nursing might include the following 10 generalizations:

1. Religious and spiritual beliefs strongly influenced Nightingale's perception of and approach to nursing. For example, the Unitarian faith to which Nightingale belonged strongly supported education [so that God's plan could be fully realized in each human being], so Nightingale focused on the development of nursing education (Montgomery, 2000).
2. Nightingale viewed her involvement in nursing as a higher calling, or vocation, and expressed the belief that other nurses should view the profession in the same way (Kalisch & Kalisch, 1995).

3. Wholism was an early and often-alluded-to concept in Nightingale's writings. For example, she consistently expressed the belief that a nurse should take into account the total environment, client, other persons, the social situation, and any other situationally related factors when providing care (Nightingale, 1859).

4. Nightingale believed that disease in general was a reparative process—nature's (or God's) effort to remedy poisoning, decay, or a reaction against conditions in which a person was placed (Nightingale, 1859).

5. "Nature" and "God" seemed to be synonymous in her writings, indicating the belief of a spiritual foundation for nursing actions based on the natural occurrence of illness (Montgomery, 2000).

6. Nightingale expressed the belief that a nurse's role was to prevent an interruption of the reparative process and to provide optimal conditions for its enhancement through careful observation and committed action to support a calm and reparative environment (Nightingale, 1859).

7. Nightingale believed that nurses should be moral agents and agents of change in society in general (Montgomery, 2000).

8. Another common theme in Nightingale's writing was that nurses should be noble, disciplined, hard-working, and selfless (Nightingale, 1859).

9. Nightingale also expressed the conviction that nurses should be independent decision makers and should provide the physician with precise facts based on sound, educated observations. For example, Nightingale believed that, in order to be effective, those seeking to provide nursing care should receive meticulous education in proper nursing techniques and approaches (Kalisch & Kalisch, 1995).

10. Finally, Nightingale expressed the thought that nursing could (and should) be a means of serving God through selfless service to mankind and that this selfless service should permeate every aspect of a nurse's existence (Montgomery, 2000).

The finished composition, or "painting," of nursing, consisting of the 10 points of color from the palette just presented might look like this: Nursing is an independent, yet parallel, profession to medicine. Nursing activities should be based on the presumption that all factors within the patient's environment influence healing. Nurses are responsible for recognizing influencing factors and correcting them so that the client's own natural healing ability progresses toward wellness. Nurses should be highly trained and educated to ensure effective care. Nurses must be dignified, of the highest moral fiber, and selfless in the performance of their work. People who choose to become nurses should do so out of a desire to serve God and humanity.

Learning Activities

1. Assess the information contained in Nightingale's theory from two different vantage points:
   - Close-up: What dots of color (ideas) are contained in this theory? List the individual ideas (dots of color) that make up the complete picture.
   - From a distance: What is the overall composition of this work? What is the "picture," or central idea, that best exemplifies the theory in general?
2. Find a visual representation (photograph, painting, line drawing, sculpture, cartoon), or create one, that expresses Nightingale's theory. Glue a copy of the image itself, or write a description of the image on page 31 to share with your classmates. Be prepared to explain why you think the image represents Nightingale's theory.
3. Find Web sites or journal articles about Nightingale and the era in which she lived and worked. Provide the URL, access date, and information about the site host. Words to use when performing a search might include:
   - Florence Nightingale
   - Victorian era
   - Crimean War
   - Nurse training schools
   - Nursing theory
4. Go to the Jones and Bartlett Web site for this text at *http://nursing.jbpub.com* and explore the Web links listed for this chapter.

Feel free to use these blank pages as a canvas for your learning activities.

Virginia Henderson's Definition of Nursing

Virginia Henderson (1897–1996) was born the fifth of eight children in Kansas City, Missouri. Because her father's law practice was located in Washington, D.C., the family moved to Virginia, where Henderson spent her childhood. Though her father was an attorney, the family did not have a great deal of money because her father's clients were primarily Native Americans in the western United States and he traveled a great deal (Eichelberger, 1991).

In 1918, Henderson entered the Army School of Nursing in Washington, D.C., graduating in 1921. Upon graduation, she became a home-visiting community health nurse, working with the Henry Street Settlement in New York City. Henderson stated that her work at the Henry Street Settlement had a significant impact on the development of her views on nursing. In 1922, Henderson began teaching nursing and 5 years later began work on a bachelor's degree and master of arts degree in nursing education at Teachers College at Columbia University. In 1930, Henderson became a faculty member at Teachers College and remained there until 1948.

While at Teachers College, Henderson became an author and researcher. Throughout her career she participated in many prestigious writing and research projects. In response to a request from the International Council of Nurses in

1960 to define nursing "independently of technology or medicine" (Henderson, 1960, rev. 1997, p. 9), Henderson created a pamphlet entitled *Basic Principles of Nursing Care*. This pamphlet was published by the International Council of Nurses in 1960 and was translated into more than 20 languages.

Henderson never married and spent her retirement years traveling. In 1991, at the age of 93, she traveled to Rome to accept an honorary award before coming before the National League for Nursing to accept yet another national award. Henderson died on March 19, 1996, at the age of 98. The Sigma Theta Tau International Library is named after her, and she left a legacy that will forever be a part of nursing theory history. Henderson has often been called the "First Lady of Nursing."

Because Henderson's definition of nursing is as true today as the day she wrote it, her booklet *Basic Principles of Nursing Care* is still in use by nurses the world over, with the most current revision being in 1997. This small book (or pamphlet, the format in which it was first created) forms the basis of a broad description of nursing; therefore, the general nature of Henderson's work roughly qualifies it as a "nursing philosophy." A quote from the introduction (Henderson, 1960, rev. 1997), written by Virginia Henderson, sums up the broad philosophical nature of Henderson's work:

> In this paper, the activities of which basic nursing is composed are outlined. Their origin in universal human needs is stressed and the nurse's continuous interpretation of the way in which these needs are modified by a particular state of the person he or she serves is shown.
>
> The intent is to describe the care that any person requires no matter what the physician's diagnosis and prescribed therapy.... The nurse's basic care [approach] is the same whether the patient is considered physically or mentally ill.... Because this booklet deals generally with nursing and is applicable to the care of any patient, it can only mention basic nursing activities.... (pp. 17–18).

Recalling the pointillism exhibited in Seurat's paintings, the palette, or points, that might make up Henderson's rendering of nursing include the following (Henderson, 1960, rev. 1997, pp. 34–35).

All humans have basic needs that include adequate functioning with respect to:

1. Breathing
2. Eating and drinking
3. Bodily elimination
4. Comfortable body postures
5. Sleeping and resting
6. Selection of proper clothing and maintenance of body temperature and skin integrity
7. Adequate cleanliness
8. Avoiding danger to self and others
9. Communicating meaningfully with others
10. Individually appropriate human developmental tasks
11. Worshipping according to one's faith
12. Work that provides a sense of accomplishment
13. Play and leisure activities
14. Opportunities to learn and satisfy curiosity

Henderson believed that:

The unique function of the nurse is to assist the individual, sick or well, in the performance of those activities contributing to health or its recovery (or to a peaceful death) that the person would perform unaided given the necessary strength, will or knowledge, and to do this in such a way as to help the individual gain independence as rapidly as possible (Henderson, 1960, rev. 1997, p. 22).

With this defining statement in mind, Henderson identified the components of basic nursing care. These components (more points of color to be added to Henderson's palette) included helping the patient, where needed, with the following (Henderson, 1960, rev. 1997, pp. 42–43):

1. Respiration
2. Eating and drinking
3. Elimination
4. Postures and ambulation
5. Sleep and rest requirements
6. Clothing needs
7. Temperature regulation
8. Hygiene
9. Avoiding danger to self and others
10. Communication, especially associated with needs and feelings

11. Religious and spiritual activities
12. The performance of appropriate work activities
13. Play and recreation
14. Learning and human developmental activities

Overall, Henderson expressed the view that a nurse's role is to follow and assist with the medical plan of care outlined by a physician and also to assume the leadership role of planning and providing basic nursing care. Nurses are independent practitioners for providing appropriate basic nursing care; however, they should not independently diagnose an ailment, prescribe medical treatment, or formulate a prognosis. The method by which the nurse facilitates optimal independence for the patient varies from patient to patient and is based on the nurse's professional judgment. Empathy coupled with knowledge and interest on the part of the nurse will enhance the healing process. The overall goal of nursing should be the promotion of as much independence as possible for the patient with regards to Henderson's 14 points.

The finished composition, or "painting," of nursing consisting of the "points of color" (information) provided might look like this: The nurse is an independent practitioner with expertise in aiding the patient to become as independent as possible in life activities. Patient independence is accomplished through appropriate medical intervention that is supported by the nurse and also by excellent basic nursing care that is formulated and carried out by the nurse autonomously. The nurse attends to the wholistic needs of the patient through educated and empathetic attention to the 14 basic needs outlined by Henderson. The nurse is an independent authority on excellent basic nursing care and also a vital aide to other practitioners in the field of health care in ensuring the provision of germane medical treatment for patients with conditions requiring it.

Learning Activities

1. Assess the information contained in this theory from two different vantage points:
   - Close-up: What dots of color (ideas) are contained in this theory? List the individual ideas (dots of color) that make up the complete picture.

- From a distance: What is the overall composition of this work? What is the "picture," or central idea, that best exemplifies the theory in general?
2. Find a visual representation (photograph, painting, line drawing, sculpture, cartoon), or create one, that expresses Henderson's theory. Glue a copy of the image itself or write a description of the image on page 38 to share with your classmates.
3. Find Web sites or journal articles about Henderson and the era in which she lived and worked. Provide the URL, access date, and information about the site host. Words to use when performing a search might include:
   - Virginia Henderson
   - Virginia Henderson International Library
   - World War I
   - The International Council of Nurses
   - Nursing theory
4. Go to the Jones and Bartlett Web site for this text at *http://nursing.jbpub.com* and explore the Web links listed for this chapter.

Feel free to use these blank pages as a canvas for your learning activities.

Ernestine Wiedenbach's Helping Art of Clinical Nursing

Ernestine Wiedenbach was born on August 18, 1900, in Hamburg, Germany, to an affluent family. As a young girl of 9, Ernestine immigrated with her family to the United States where she became interested in becoming a nurse after observing a private duty nurse take care of her ailing grandmother. Wiedenbach completed a bachelor of arts degree at Wellesley College in 1922 and then entered the Johns Hopkins School of Nursing shortly thereafter. After completing her nursing degree at Johns Hopkins in 1925, Wiedenbach worked in many different areas of nursing, including hospital bedside, public health, and administrative nursing. Wiedenbach completed a master's degree and certificate in public health nursing at Teachers College, Columbia University, in 1934. She eventually became a professional nurse writer for the *American Journal of Nursing*. At age 45, Wiedenbach enrolled in the School for Midwives at the Maternity Center Association of New York. After graduating with a degree in midwifery in 1946, Wiedenbach practiced as a nurse midwife and taught evening courses at Teachers College until 1951. Wiedenbach taught at Yale School of Nursing and helped start a master's degree program where she directed the maternal-newborn program. Wiedenbach also continued to publish, writing a textbook in 1958 about family-centered maternity nursing and another in 1964 entitled *Clinical Nursing: A Helping Art*. Wiedenbach retired in 1966 (Tomey & Alligood, 2002). She is probably most well known for her work in theory development and maternal-child nursing. She never married and died at the age of 97 on March 8, 1998 (Guide to Ernestine Wiedenbach papers, Yale University, retrieved on May 28, 2003, from *http://webtext.library.yale.edu/xml2html/mssa.1647 .con.html#top*).

Wiedenbach asserted that there are four elements to clinical nursing:

1. *Philosophy*: An attitude toward life and reality that evolves from each nurse's beliefs and code of conduct. Philosophy motivates the nurse to act, guides thinking about what to do, and influences decision making (Tomey & Alligood, 2002). According to Wiedenbach, a nursing philosophy has three essential components (George, 2002):
   a. Reverence for the gift of life
   b. Respect for the dignity, worth, autonomy, and individuality of each human being
   c. A resolution to act on personally and professionally held beliefs
2. *Purpose*: That which the nurse wants to accomplish through what he or she does—the overall goals for professional practice, including activities directed toward the overall good of the patient (Tomey & Alligood, 2002).
3. *Practice*: Observable nursing actions that are influenced by disciplined thoughts and feelings toward meeting the patient's need for help. These actions are goal directed and patient centered (Tomey & Alligood, 2002).
4. *Art*: The art of clinical nursing consists of (Tomey & Alligood, 2002):
   a. The nurse's understanding of the patient's condition, situation, and need.
   b. The nurse's internal goals and external actions that are meant to enhance patient capability through appropriate nursing care.
   c. The nurse's activities directed toward improvement of the patient's condition through artful utilization of the medical plan of care.
   d. The nurse's interventions aimed at prevention of recurrence of the current concern or development of a new concern.

Additionally, Wiedenbach further defined her vision of what nursing is in a global sense by defining key terms commonly used to refer to nursing practice. These definitions themselves do not fully define the profession; however, nurses often use global terms such as "patient," "helping," "knowledge," and "nursing action" to loosely describe what they do. In specifically defining what each of these terms means within the context of her theory, Wiedenbach imparts clarity and power to her work and sets the stage for productive exploration and debate.

It may initially seem that definitions for commonly used words or phrases are unnecessary because everyone probably knows what they mean (we are all nurses, right?). However, this is not necessarily the case. Often, such global terms do not mean the same thing to individual nurses or to subgroups within the profession. When two or more nurses discuss nursing within the context of various environments (e.g., when giving and taking report in the hospital, engaging in academic debates or creating written papers in school, or reading and producing published material found in professional journals), they may *think* that they are in total agreement about the meanings of basic terminology, when in fact, they are not. For instance, during a change of shift report, the *reporting* nurse might refer to "excessive stimulus" of a patient and mean to indicate that there were too many relatives in the room visiting all day, whereas the nurse *receiving* the report may construe this to mean that the patient is demonstrating symptoms of internal neurological overstimulation caused by a pathological medical condition. The only way to truly understand what is meant by use of the term "excessive stimulus" is to clarify the definition of the term from the reporting nurse's perspective.

Words are easy to misunderstand, and they are powerful in shaping perceptions, so it is important to carefully define terminology. Here are five terms, defined by Wiedenbach, that elucidate the overall meaning of her theory and clarify what the theory means in terms of actual nursing practice (Tomey & Alligood, 2002):

1. The *patient* is any person who has entered the healthcare system and is receiving help of some kind, such as care, teaching, or advice. The patient need not be ill; someone receiving health-related education would qualify as a patient.
2. A *need for help* is defined as any measure desired by the patient that has the potential to restore or extend the patient's ability to cope with various life situations that affect health and wellness.
3. [Clinical] *judgment* represents the nurse's likeliness to make sound decisions. Sound decisions are based on differentiating fact from assumption and relating them to cause and effect. Sound *judgment* is the result

of disciplined functioning of mind and emotions and improves with expanded knowledge and increased clarity of professional purpose.

4. Nursing *skills* are carried out to achieve a specific patient-centered purpose, rather than completion of the skill itself being the end goal. *Skills* are made up of a variety of actions and characterized by harmony of movement, precision, and effective use of self.

5. Each *person* (whether nurse or patient) is endowed with a unique potential to develop self-sustaining resources. People generally tend toward independence and fulfillment of responsibilities. Self-awareness and self-acceptance are essential to personal integrity and self-worth. Whatever an individual does at any given moment represents the best available judgment for that person at the time.

Wiedenbach describes nursing in a global sense as effective identification of a patient's need for help through observation of presenting behaviors and symptoms, exploration of the *meaning* of those symptoms with the patient, and codetermining the cause(s) of discomfort. The patient's ability to resolve the discomfort is then assessed, and help from the nurse or other healthcare professionals is provided as needed.

The finished composition, or "painting," of nursing consisting of the "points of color" (information) just provided might look like this: Nursing primarily consists of identifying a patient's need for help. If the need for help requires intervention, the nurse facilitates the medical plan of care and also creates and enacts a nursing plan of care based on individual needs and expressed desires of the patient. In providing care, a nurse exercises sound judgment through deliberative, practiced, and educated recognition of sentinel symptoms. The patient's perception of the situation is an important consideration to the nurse when providing competent care. Nurses respect the individuality, dignity, worth, and autonomy of each patient and understand that patients generally value independence. When assessing a patient's need for help and resulting response to care, it is important to remember that human beings generally do the best they can with what they have (emotionally, physically, intellectually, socially), making the best judgments possible *for them*, at any given moment. Need for help, and the resulting care provided, is more important than attempting to determine and/or judge *why* a patient may have made a particular life decision.

Learning Activities

1. Assess the information contained in this theory from two different vantage points:
   - Close-up: What dots of color (ideas) are contained in this theory? List the individual ideas (dots of color) that make up the complete picture.
   - From a distance: What is the overall composition of this work? What is the "picture," or central idea, that best exemplifies the theory in general?
2. Find a visual representation (photograph, painting, line drawing, sculpture, cartoon), or create one, that expresses Wiedenbach's theory. Glue a copy of the image itself or write a description of the image on page 46 to share with your classmates.
3. Find Web sites or journal articles about Wiedenbach and her theory. Words to use when performing a search might include:
   - Ernestine Wiedenbach
   - Nursing theory
   - The Prescriptive Theory of Nursing
   - The Helping Art of Nursing
4. Go to the Jones and Bartlett Web site for this text at *http://nursing.jbpub.com* and explore the Web links listed for this chapter.

Feel free to use these blank pages as a canvas for your learning activities.

Jean Watson's Theory of Human/Transpersonal Caring

Jean Watson was born in a small, close-knit town in the Appalachian Mountains of West Virginia in the 1940s. Watson graduated from the Lewis Gale School of Nursing in Roanoke, West Virginia, in 1961. After marrying, Watson moved to her husband Doug's home state of Colorado, where she gave birth to two daughters. She continued her nursing studies at the University of Colorado, earning a B.S. in 1964, an M.S. in psychiatric and mental health nursing in 1966, and a Ph.D. in educational psychology and counseling in 1973. Watson then joined the nursing faculty at the University of Colorado Health Sciences Center and served in many teaching and administrative roles, including chair and assistant dean of the undergraduate nursing program, director of the doctoral program, and dean of the School of Nursing. Watson was instrumental in creating the Center for Human Caring at the University of Colorado. This center was created to develop and use knowledge of human caring and healing in nursing and to assist in efforts to transform the healthcare system into a more care-centered entity. Watson lives in Boulder, Colorado, and continues to function as a part of the nursing faculty at the University of Colorado in the capacity of Distinguished Professor of Nursing and holds the Murchinson-Scoville Endowed Chair in Caring Science (Tomey & Alligood, 2002).

In the following passage, Watson discusses the development of her Theory of Human Caring (retrieved on May 1, 2003, from *http://www.uchsc.edu/nursing/caring*):

> The Theory of Human Caring was developed between 1975–1979, while engaged in teaching at the University of Colorado; it emerged from my own views of nursing, combined and informed by my doctoral studies in educational-clinical and social psychology. It was my initial attempt to bring meaning and focus to nursing as an emerging discipline and distinct health profession with its own unique values, knowledge and practices, with its own ethic and mission to society. The work also was influenced by my involvement with an integrated academic nursing curriculum and efforts to find common meaning and order to nursing that transcended settings, populations, specialty, subspecialty areas, and so forth.
>
> From my emerging perspective, I tried to make explicit nursing's values, knowledge, and practices of human caring that are geared toward subjective inner healing processes and the life world of the experiencing person, requiring unique caring-healing arts and a framework called "carative factors," which complemented conventional medicine, but stood in stark contrast to "curative factors." At the same time, this emerging philosophy and theory of human caring sought to balance the cure orientation of medicine, giving nursing its unique disciplinary, scientific, and professional standing with itself and its public.

Watson indicates throughout her work that all human beings have an inherent need to participate in caring exchanges, both as giver and receiver, and that nursing holds the essence of this fundamental need.

Because Watson communicates her theory with such clarity, and because the central theme of "care" resonates with so many nurses throughout the world, Watson's Theory of Human/Transpersonal Caring has become a theoretical mainstay for many individual nurses, and also entire nursing education programs in the United States and around the world.

The major elements that constitute Watson's continually evolving theory are:

- Clinical caritas processes (the term *caritas* comes from a Greek term meaning to cherish, appreciate, give special attention to, and value as precious)

- Transpersonal caring relationships
- Caring moments/caring occasions

Other dynamic aspects of the theory that are emerging include:

- *Expanded views of self and person* (nurse and client awareness of transpersonal "mindbodyspirit" with unity of being and recognition of embodied spirit)
- *Caring–healing consciousness* (nurse's cultivated intention to care and to promote healing)
- *Caring consciousness* (state of being within the caring exchange mindfully, and recognizing the distinct energy within the caring moment)
- Recognition of the *wholeness and connectedness* of all
- Being open to the belief that a*dvanced caring–healing modalities/nursing arts* constitute a valid future model for the advanced practice of nursing, consciously guided by one's theoretical–philosophical orientation

Here is a closer look at the first major element of Watson's theory, the 10 clinical caritas processes. A genuine caring exchange between nurse and client is possible when the nurse mindfully enacts these caring processes (Watson, 2003):

1. Practice of loving-kindness and equanimity within the context of an intentional caring consciousness.
2. Being authentically present.
3. Cultivation of one's own spiritual practices and transpersonal self, going beyond ego self.
4. Developing and sustaining a helping-trusting, authentic caring relationship.
5. Being present to, and supportive of, the expression of positive and negative feelings as a connection with deeper spirit of self and the one being cared for.
6. Creative use of self and all ways of knowing as part of the caring process; to engage in artistry of caring-healing practices.
7. Engaging in genuine teaching-learning experience that attends to unity of being and meaning, while attempting to stay within other's frame of reference.
8. Creating a healing environment at all levels (physical as well as nonphysical, subtle environment of energy and consciousness), whereby wholeness, beauty, comfort, dignity, and peace are potentiated.

9. Assisting with basic needs, with an intentional caring consciousness, administering human care essentials, which potentiate alignment of mindbodyspirit, wholeness, and unity of being in all aspects of care; tending to both embodied spirit and evolving spiritual emergence of both other and self.

10. Opening and attending to spiritual-mysterious and existential dimensions of one's own life-death; soul care for self and the one being cared for.

These 10 caring processes outline a nursing practice whereby it is recognized by the nurse that all of life is interconnected. Each nurse–client exchange is made up of shared energy between all who are present during the interaction. The nurse is called to not only recognize the evolving physical/spiritual being in the client being cared for, but to also recognize and nurture the physical/spiritual being in the self, for one cannot provide authentic caring to another without first being able to care for the self.

The second major element of Watson's theory is *transpersonal caring relationship*. Transpersonal caring relationships are the foundation of nursing work. Transpersonal caring seeks to connect with and embrace the spirit or soul of the other through the processes of caring and healing and being in authentic relation, in the moment (Watson, 2003). Transpersonal caring implies that the nurse consciously focuses on the uniqueness of self, other, and the present moment, wherein the nurse/client exchange is mutual and reciprocal, each fully embodied in the moment, while paradoxically capable of transcending the moment and opening to new possibilities. Transpersonal caring calls for personal reflection and an ability on the part of the nurse to be mindfully present to self and others. The transpersonal nurse has the ability to center consciousness and intentionality on caring, healing, and wholeness, rather than on disease, illness, and pathology. The nurse attempts to enter into and stay within the other's frame of reference for connecting with the inner life world of meaning and spirit of the other. Together they join in a mutual search for meaning and wholeness. The authentic transpersonal caring exchange will potentiate comfort measures, pain control, a sense of well-being, wholeness, and/or even spiritual transcendence of suffering. The person is viewed as whole and complete, regardless of illness or disease (Watson, 2003).

The third major element of Watson's theory is *caring moments/caring occasions*. A caring occasion occurs whenever the nurse and patient come together with their unique life histories and phenomenal fields in a human-to-human transaction. The coming together in a given moment becomes a focal point in space and time. It becomes transcendent, whereby experience and perception take place, but the actual caring occasion has a greater field of its own in a given moment. The process goes beyond itself, yet arises from aspects of itself that become part of the life history of each person, as well as part of some larger, more complex pattern of life (Watson, 1988). A caring moment consists of actions and choices made by both the nurse and patient. The moment of coming together presents each with the opportunity to decide how to participate in the relationship. If the caring moment is transpersonal, the client and nurse feel connected with one another at the spiritual level, thus the moments in the interaction transcend time and space and open up new possibilities for healing and human connection at a deeper level than physical, social, or verbal interaction (Watson, 2003).

In summary, Watson's theory is about mindful, in-the-moment, committed caring for both self and patient. One of the rewards of enacting Watson's theory in daily nursing practice is deeper knowledge, understanding of, and compassion for self and others. Watson writes:

> we learn from one another how to be human by identifying ourselves with others, [and] finding their dilemmas in ourselves. What we all learn from it is self-knowledge. The self we learn about.... is every self. IT is universal—the human self. We learn to recognize ourselves in others.... [this kind of interaction] keeps alive our common humanity and avoids reducing self or other to the moral status of object (Watson, 1988, pp. 59–60).

The finished composition, or "painting," of nursing, consisting of the "points of color" from the palette of information contained in Watson's theory might look like this: Nursing primarily consists of a core of intentional caring, intertwined with excellent nursing skills. The nurse and patient are equally valued in the nurse–patient interaction, with both contributing various attributes to the caring environment. Central to excellent transpersonal caring on the part of the nurse is the realization that connections between patient and nurse exist on many levels, from the overt physical environment to deep levels of energy exchange that are not readily observable in the traditional sense. Spirituality, intentionality, and mindful attention to the here and now within the human-to-human exchange enables the nurse to wholistically express caring in the physical, emotional, psychological, spiritual, social, and matter/energy realms simultaneously.

Envision rainbows of light particles surrounding and enveloping the nurse and patient. These particles are vibrating, intermingling, ebbing, and flowing as the transpersonal moment occurs. At close proximity, individual colors emitted by both the patient and the nurse intensify and mix, and when the two move away from each other the colors soften and become pale. When nurse and patient conclude the interaction, and one or the other moves increasingly away, there is a pale trail of vibrating color that follows each participant, with lingering hues of the nurse within the client and the client within the nurse.

Jean Watson: Personal Experience and Background in Being a Nurse Theorist

One never expects, or at least I never expected, nor anticipated, being a so-called nurse theorist. It happened gradually and indirectly, along the way, via a process of scholarly writing in my efforts to make sense of nursing. My journey began as a process of exploring deep meaning, integrity, distinction, and philosophical underpinning of the nature of nursing. This exploration was influenced by having a background in psychiatric mental health nursing and having completed my Ph.D., studying various existential and phenomenological aspects of human existence. These experiences allowed me the privilege of examining the diverse theories or personality, ways of being in the world, and exploring various views of humanity, dynamics of human behavior, and so on.

Writing my first book was also a healing experience for me personally, in that I had just joined the faculty of the University of Colorado and was distressed that most of the focus and direction for advancing nursing was within the context of medical science, technology, and conventional research related to disease treatment and curing, almost at all costs.

Thus, after completing my Ph.D. and drawing upon my intellectual and educational clinical experiences and my masters degree in psychiatric-mental health nursing, my journey began more formally. My first book, Nursing: The Philosophy and Science of Caring (1979, 1985), was triggered by my new academic world entry and critique of status quo with medical focus on nursing. It began my exploration of core values, knowledge, and context for nursing science, with its focus on humanity and human caring, healing, human experiences, and health in contrast with, but complementary to medical science. It offered a philosophical and scientific-research orientation, as well as a language and structure for the phenomenon of human caring.

In this first work, I was asking myself the question, "Is there a core of nursing that transcends medical cure approaches and clinical settings, diagnoses, treatments, and so on, that relates to what nursing offers to humanity?" Further, I was questioning whether there is a core of nursing that is universal and timeless that is not defined by tasks and skills and actions that nurses do, while pursuing a framework of human caring that defines nursing and its contribution to society, beyond medicine and medical science.

That same personal exploratory process of mine acknowledged that the current state of nursing was void of a meaningful philosophical foundation for its model of science. Therefore, my first book offered a personal answer to my own quest/questioning and served as a treatise and guide for defining and advancing nursing for its future, while honoring, identifying, and naming nurses and nursing's timeless and ancient gift to humankind. Further, I wanted to acknowledge to nursing and the public the essential nature of nursing's role in human caring, health, and well-being, which needs to be sustained and advanced if human caring is to evolve and survive in the world. It was a decade or so later that my work began to be considered a theory and be discovered as a meaningful philosophical-theoretical framework for nursing.

Personal Views of Being a Nurse Theorist

On a more personal level, especially because my work has been studied and explored via professional practice models, empirical validation through research, and educational curricular models, I have received offers of remarkable learning experiences around the world. My studies and contact with students, faculty, and clinicians have included every continent; I have been around the world at least 12 times, touching the hearts and lives and minds of nurses in hospitals, educational programs, and diverse clinical settings.

Likewise, these many thousands of nurses have expanded and deeply touched my mind, heart, and life by helping to affirm and extend my own thinking and scholarship. My latest work has evolved as a model of caring science, which provides a framework both for nursing and beyond nursing, allowing diverse theories to be explored and located within a shared worldview. Caring science unites and seeks converging ideas and models, within a unitary worldview and ethic of belonging to an infinite field of universal love, which holds the world and humanity in a global field (Levinas, 1969; Watson, 2005).

My work also requires personal practices of my own theory in order to sustain authenticity and dynamic evolution, constantly changing toward more depth and wisdom, beyond knowledge per se. Thus, my first *caritas* process, *cultivation of loving kindness and equanimity toward self and other*, requires my engagement as well as acknowledging such basic practices for self, in order to sustain humanistic altruistic values and authentic caring presence and relationship with others. Thus, I still am trying to catch up with my own theory, because it is larger and deeper than my own knowledge, but an ongoing personal, spiritual journey toward inner life world of self, honoring the deep subjective inner life world of self/other. This personal/professional practice seeks to "see" who is the spirit-filled person behind the physical appearance, behind the diagnosis and treatment, behind the behavior I/we may not like or approve. This reminds me and others that one person's level of humanity reflects on the other, and therefore, caring theory is an ongoing dynamic process of understanding life and all the vicissitudes of human existence, from birth to death and beyond—seeking wisdom, compassion, love, and personal integration of knowledge and all of life's known and unknown experiences. This work embraces mystery, humility, and surrender, while trusting in deep love and one's soul journey on the Earth plane.

Other Personal Notes

My life experiences and own personal tragedies/blessings have been my teachers and also influenced my writings and theory expansions. For example, having a serious traumatic eye injury several years ago allowed me the gift of receiving and experiencing my own theory of caring from my husband. I had to be still for almost 3 months, with only 15-minute breaks, lying face down on a massage table, allowing for the eye to heal. This time of stillness and quiet contemplation awakened a deeper appreciation of life and all the small things we take for granted. Further, my own theory guided my approach to my care. Rituals, beauty, nature, meditation, music/sound, silence, and intentional loving touch therapies and massage were incorporated into my caring. No negative energy, such as television or newspapers, was allowed into my healing space; people took off their shoes when they entered the room. Poetry and literature and healing cards were read to me. I was given full body massages; I dwelled in silence and contemplative time for meditation. I was grateful for everything and life itself; I treasured listening to sounds of nature and using a mirror to look outside my window, even upside down, to see the trees, sky, and birds. I wrote psalms as a meditative and sacred act of expression and release (Watson, 1999).

I cherished basic daily living activities and engaged in meditation and praying without ceasing, as a way to sustain myself and my emotional, psychic, and physical pain. All of these experiences, painful and otherwise, both validated and affirmed my theory of caring and healing, while allowing me the privilege of experiencing it from the inside out. These and other experiences provided more personal/professional confidence and courage related to my philosophies and theory, leading to my book, *Caring Science as Sacred Science* (2005). This book acknowledged the sacredness of all of nursing, in that we are dealing with the life force and mystery of life itself.

Other personal practices that continue to inform my work and writings include exposure to nurses in many other cultures; these global cultural human experiences help me to appreciate and deepen my understanding of the universality of human conditions and the timeless need for human caring and healing. Such knowledge, wisdom, and insights go beyond conventional medical-scientific approaches that often restrict nurses in their education and practices and learning of human caring, healing, and health.

More recently I am blessed to be working with many hospitals, nurses, and other staff to deepen and sustain human caring theory as a living intellectual model of authentic heart-centered practices of *caritas* nursing and health care—restoring love and caring as the foundation for healing self and other, thus transforming self and systems. Such experiments and pilot programs are seeking criteria to designate hospitals as authentic caring science institutions, not confined to medical-techno-cure focus, rather returning to caring and love as the core of healing and healing environments. Thus, my personal professional journey continues to intersect, as the personal becomes the professional, in a living model of caring science.

Most recently my work is culminating and continuing through Watson Caring Science Institute, a nonprofit foundation, created in 2007 to extend and deepen caring science work in the world. The foundation's Web site is at www.watsoncaringscience.org. The latest project is acknowledging to the public that nurses and nursing stand as an archetype for human caring and love to humanity. This project is designed to reach a million nurses, meditating at the same time, to radiate a global caring field to humanity around the world; this project coincides with the international year of the nurse in 2010. The global caring field meditation project began January 1, 2010, at noon, wherever anyone was in the world. The global caring field meditation is scheduled to be repeated on May 12, 2010, which is Florence Nightingale's birthday and her centenary year. It concludes on December 31, 2010, yet extends into 2011 with the Hiroshima International Conference on Caring and Peace, making new connections between the nurse's role in sustaining human caring and affirming the relationship between caring and peace in the world.

Finally, the work in caring science allows for a full maturation of nursing as a distinct discipline and profession in its own right, offering wisdom, vision, and sustaining directions for the future of caring and healing for humanity, and its evolution toward a moral community of global caring, healing, and health for all.

Key Background Representative Books

Bevis, E. O., & Watson, J. (1989). *Toward a caring curriculum: A new pedagogy for nursing.* New York: National League for Nursing.

Bevis, E. O., & Watson, J. (2000, reprinted). *Toward a caring curriculum. A new pedagogy for nursing.* Sudbury, MA: Jones and Bartlett.

Chinn, P., & Watson, J. (Eds.). (1994). *Art and aesthetics of nursing.* New York: National League for Nursing.

Leininger, M., & Watson, J. (Eds.). (1990). *The caring imperative in education.* New York: National League for Nursing.

Taylor, R., & Watson, J. (Eds.). (1989). *They shall not hurt: Human suffering and human caring.* Boulder, CO: University Press of Colorado.

Watson, J. (Ed.). (1994). *Applying the art and science of human caring.* New York: National League for Nursing.

Watson, J. (1999). *Nursing: Human science and human care* (3rd ed.). New York: Appleton-Century-Crofts. New York: NLN (Jones and Bartlett).

Watson, J. (1999). *Postmodern nursing and beyond.* Edinburgh, Scotland, UK: Churchill Livingstone/W. B. Saunders.

Watson, J. (2002). *Assessing and measuring caring in nursing and health sciences.* New York: Springer.

Watson, J. (2007). Reconsidering nursing education scholarship. In U. Zeitler (Ed.), *Center for innovation in nursing education.* Aarhus, Denmark: The Center for Innovation in Nursing Education.

Watson, J. (2008). *Assessing and measuring caring in nursing and health sciences* (2nd rev. ed.). New York: Springer.

Watson, J. (2008). *Nursing. The philosophy and science of caring* (Revised and updated ed.). Boulder, CO: University Press of Colorado.

Watson, J., & Ray, M. (Eds.). (1988). *The ethics of care and the ethics of cure: Synthesis in chronicity.* New York: National League for Nursing.

Key Background Representative Journal Articles

(* = Refereed journal)

*Cowling, R., Smith, M., Watson, J., & Newman, M. (2008). The power of wholeness, consciousness, and caring. A dialogue on nursing science, art and healing. *Advances in Nursing Science, 31*(1), E41–E51.

*Fawcett, J. (2002). The nurse theorists: 21st century updates—Jean Watson. *Nursing Science Quarterly, 15*(3), 214–219.

*Fawcett, J., Watson, J., Neuman, B., & Hinton-Walker, P. (2001). On theories and evidence. *Journal of Nursing Scholarship, 33*(2), 121–128.

*Foster, R. (contributor). (2007). Tribute to the theorists: Jean Watson over the years. *Nursing Science Quarterly, 20*(1), 7.

*Hemsley, M. S., Glass, N., & Watson, J. (2006). Taking the eagle's view: Using Watson's conceptual model to investigate the extraordinary and transformative experiences of nurse healers. *Journal of Holistic Nursing Practice, 20*(2), 85–94.

*Johns, C., & Watson, J. (Eds.). (1999). Reflective caring practices [Guest editorial]. *International Journal of Human Caring, 3*(2), 5–7.

*Persky, G., Nelson, J.W., Watson, J., & Bent, K. (2008). Profile of a nurse effective in caring. *Nursing Administration Quarterly, 32*(1), 15–20.

*Quinn, J. F., Smith, M., Ritenbaugh, C., Swanson, K., & Watson, M. J. (2003). Research guidelines for assessing the impact of the healing relationship in clinical nursing. *Alternative Therapies in Health and Medicine, 9*(Suppl. 3), A65–A79.

*Watson, J. (1998). Nightingale and the enduring legacy of transpersonal human caring. *Journal of Holistic Nursing, 16*(2), 292–294.

*Watson, J. (2000). Leading via caring-healing: The four-fold way toward transformative leadership. *Nursing Administration Quarterly, 25*(1), 1–6.

*Watson, J. (2000). Postmodern nursing: Revisioning nursing's transpersonal caring. *Hong Kong Nursing Journal, 36*(4), 31–33.

*Watson, J. (2000). Reconsidering caring in the home. *Journal of Geriatric Nursing, 21*(6), 330–331.

*Watson, J. (2000). Via negativa: Considering caring by way of non-caring. *Australian Journal of Holistic Nursing, 7*(1), 4–8.

*Watson, J. (2001). Post-hospital nursing: Shortages, shifts, and scripts. *Nursing Administrative Quarterly, 25*(3), 77–82.

*Watson, J. (2002). Caring and healing our living and dying. *The International Nurse, 15*(2), 4–5.

*Watson, J. (2002). Holistic nursing and caring: A values based approach. *Journal of Japan Academy of Nursing Science, 22*(2), 69–74.

*Watson, J. (2002). Intentionality and caring-healing consciousness: A theory of transpersonal nursing. *Holistic Nursing Practice, 16*(4), 12–19.

*Watson, J. (2002). Metaphysics of virtual caring communities. *International Journal of Human Caring, 6*(1), 41–45.

*Watson, J. (2002, Spring). Nursing: Seeking its source and survival [Guest editorial]. *ICU NURS WEB Journal, 9,* 1–7. Retrieved from www.nursing.gr/J.W.editorial.pdf

*Watson, J. (2003). Love and caring: Ethics of face and hand. *Nursing Administration Quarterly, 27*(3), 197–202.

*Watson, J. (2004). *Caritas* and *communitas*: An ethic for caring science. *Journal Japan Academy of Nursing Science, 24*(1), 66–71.

*Watson, J. (2004). The relational core of nursing as partnership [Invited commentary]. *Journal of Advanced Nursing, 47*(3), 241–250.

*Watson, J. (2005). Caring science: Belonging before being as ethical cosmology. *Nursing Science Quarterly, 18*(4), 4–5.

*Watson, J. (2005). Commentary on Shattell, M. (2004). Nurse-patient interaction: A review of the literature. *Journal of Clinical Nursing, 14,* 530–532.

*Watson, J. (2005). Current issues and haunting concerns for survival of nursing profession. *Japanese Journal of Nursing Science, 30*(11), 50–53.

Watson, J. (2005). Love and caring [Reposted]. *Alternative Journal of Nursing, 9.* Retrieved January 12, 2010, from http://www.altjn.com/perspectives/love_caring.pdf

Watson, J. (2005). An overview of Watson's theory of human caring. *Bulletin of Japanese Red Cross University College of Nursing, 19,* 2005.

*Watson, J. (2005). What may I ask, is happening to nursing knowledge and professional practices? What is nursing thinking at this turn in human history? [Editorial]. *Journal of Clinical Nursing, 14,* 913–914.

*Watson, J. (2006). Can an ethic of caring be maintained? *Journal of Advanced Nursing, 54*(3), 257–259.

*Watson, J. (2006). Carative factors—*Caritas* processes guide to professional nursing. *Danish Clinical Nursing Journal, 20*(3), 21–27l.

*Watson, J. (2006). Caring theory as ethical guide to administrative and clinical practices. *Nursing Administrative Quarterly, 30*(1), 48–55.

Watson, J. (2006). Caring theory as ethical guide to administrative and clinical practices. *JONA'S healthcare law, ethics, and regulation, 8*(1), 87–83. [(Reprinted from

Watson, J. (2006). Caring theory as ethical guide to administrative and clinical practices. *Nursing Administrative Quarterly, 30*(1), 48–55)].

*Watson, J. (2006). Frontline and backstage caring: American nurse/world-wide nurses. *American Nurse Today, 1*(1), 24–28.

*Watson, J. (2006). Spiritual pilgrimage as *caritas* action in the world. *Journal of Holistic Nursing, 24*(4), 289–296.

*Watson, J. (2007). Theoretical questions and concerns: Responses from a caring science framework. *Nursing Science Quarterly, 20*(1), 13–15.

*Watson, J. (2007). Watson's theory of human caring and subjective living experiences: Disciplinary guide to professional nursing practice. *Brazilian Clinical Nursing Journal: Texto and Contexto, 16*(1), 129–135.

*Watson, J. (2008). Social justice and caring: A model of caring science as a hopeful paradigm for moral justice for humanity. *Creative Nursing: A Journal of Values, Issues, Experience & Collaboration, 14*(22), 54–61.

*Watson, J. (2009). Caring science and human caring theory: Transforming personal/professional practices in nursing and healthcare. *Journal of Health and Human Services Administration, 31*(4, symposium issue), 466–482.

*Watson, J. (2009). Concept of caring from Watson's perspective. *Nursing Science Quarterly, 22*(3).

*Watson, J. (2009). From theory to practice: Caring science according to Watson and Brewer. *Nursing Science Quarterly, 22*(4), 339–345.

*Watson, J., Bauer, R., & Biley, F. (2002). Bavarian nursing secret: An inside view. *Reflections on Nursing Leadership: Sigma Theta Tau International Magazine, 28*(1), 26–28.

*Watson, J., Biley, F. C., & Biley, A. M. (2002). Aesthetics, postmodern nursing, complementary therapies and more: An Internet dialogue. *Complementary Therapies in Nursing and Midwifery, 8*, 81–83.

*Watson, J., & Foster, R. (2003). The attending nurse caring model: Integrating theory, evidence and advanced caring-healing therapeutics for transforming professional practice. *Journal of Clinical Nursing, 12*, 360–365.

Watson, J., & Smith, M. C. (2002). Caring science and the science of unitary human beings: A trans-theoretical discourse for nursing knowledge development. *Journal of Advanced Nursing, 37*(5), 452–461.

Learning Activities

1. Assess the information contained in this theory from two different vantage points:

   - Close-up: What dots of color (ideas) are contained in this theory? List the individual ideas (dots of color) that make up the complete picture.

   - From a distance: What is the overall composition of this work? What is the "picture," or central idea, that best exemplifies the theory in general?

2. Find a visual representation (photograph, painting, line drawing, sculpture, cartoon), or create one, that expresses Watson's theory. Glue a copy of the image itself or write a description of the image on page 63 to share with your classmates.

3. Find Web sites about Watson's theory or locate journal articles about her life and theories. Words to use when performing a search might include:
   • Jean Watson
   • Theory of Human Caring
   • Nursing theory
   • Alternative therapies

4. Go to the Jones and Bartlett Web site for this text at *http://nursing.jbpub.com* and explore the Web links listed for this chapter.

5. Compare and contrast the similarities and differences among the four nurses who have given us the nursing philosophies described in Part II. How are they alike personally, professionally, conceptually, and ideally? How are they different? What makes each unique? What part do you think their differences played in the development of each unique nursing philosophy?

6. If you could ask any one of the four theorists discussed in Part II one question, which theorist would you ask, what would you ask them, and why would you want to know?

Feel free to use these blank pages as a canvas for your learning activities.

Theories about
Broad Nursing Practice Areas:
Grand Theories

PART
III

Envisioning Theories Through Mandala Art

The purpose of a *grand theory* is to organize various pieces of information around an identified broad concept, or central point, associated with nursing practice. This is done so that other nurses may better understand the individual components that influence nursing perceptions and practices connected to a specific concept. For example, nurses routinely discuss issues surrounding "health" and "wellness" when providing care in a wide range of settings. Different nurses may have dissimilar perceptions about what factors influence or determine states of "health" and "wellness." These differences may dramatically affect how nursing care is delivered by individual nurses; thus it becomes useful to formally explore and clarify the terms "health" and "wellness" so that nurses, as a group, may productively use, discuss, and investigate these important concepts.

In art, mandalas are forms in which there is a central, or focal, point around which multiple symmetrically arranged elements exist. In mandalas, there are an infinite number of patterns that may be formed around an infinite number of unique focal points. Mandalas are abundant in nature, appearing for example, in human cells, snowflakes, flowers, the iris of the eye, spider webs, whirlpools, and tornados. All have a center point around which multiple elements are arranged, creating unity and completeness. Throughout history, human beings in all cultures have recognized mandalas in nature and have sought to create their own mandalas to visually represent uniquely human interests. Even today,this ancient art form has many enthusiasts, as evidenced by the existence of numerous mandala artists, books, clubs, and Web sites, which are accessed by thousands of people around the world every day. Color Plate 10.1, found in the color insert section of this text, shows a picture from a Web site where people share personal mandala art creations.

Here are other representations of mandalas used throughout the world:

- Many Christian cathedrals throughout Europe have labyrinths. Labyrinths are similar to mandalas in that they have a central point around which symmetrically arranged elements form a balanced pattern, in some form or another, on the floors, walls, and ceilings. Many believe that walking a labyrinth, or tracing the outline of a smaller one with a finger or stylus, induces a calm meditative state wherein the order, unity, and beauty of the universe may be contemplated. Amiens Cathedral in France was completed around 1289 (see Color Plates 10.2 and 10.3 in the color insert). This cathedral has a tile labyrinth on the floor (Color Plate 10.2) on which hundreds of visitors a year contemplatively walk the lines that form the design (Color Plate 10.3).
- Mandalas can be seen in most Christian cathedrals all over the world in the form of rose windows (Color Plate 10.4 in the color insert), or other decorative designs such as the one found in the bottom of a baptismal font (Color Plate 10.5 in the color insert). Both photos are from the Cathedral of the Madeline in Salt Lake City, Utah.
- In the Buddhist tradition, intricate sand mandalas are created, viewed for a short time, and then swept away to represent the cycle of life and rebirth, and also to represent the impermanence of all things. The sand mandala shown in Color Plate 10.6 (in the color insert) was created in June of 2003 at the Philadelphia Museum of Art by the Venerable Losang Samten.
- The mandala form is also evident in English, Asian, and Greek gardens, as evidenced by a contemporary garden in Canada (Color Plate 10.7 in the color insert).

Mandalas are useful in illustrating the concept of *grand theories* in nursing because, like grand theories, mandalas contain a central point of interest surrounded by smaller components symmetrically organized into a unified work. Like grand theories, mandalas are purposely arranged to provide beauty and clarity. Both have distinct boundaries meant to provide a sense of unity and completeness; however, the symmetry of the design easily allows for the inclusion of additional layers without significantly altering the central point.

When reading about theories that contain a broad, central point of interest, systematically surrounded by supporting or explanatory concepts, envision a mandala and ask these 10 questions:

1. What is the central point around which all of the smaller concepts cluster?
2. What are the names of the smaller concepts?
3. Where do the smaller concepts fall in relation to the central concept?
4. Envision whether a smaller concept is closely related to the central concept, thereby belonging close to the center of the design or if it is a more loosely connected concept that would belong on the periphery of the design.
5. Would the central concept be large, occupying most of the space in the overall design, or smaller, with the supporting components occupying most of the space?
6. Are there many small components of equal size, or would there be some components that are significantly larger than others?
7. Would the theory form a smooth, circular design, or a linear, angular design?
8. Would the completed design appear cluttered or sparse with regards to number, size, and spacing of central and peripheral elements?
9. Would the peripheral margins of the design be open or closed?
10. What colors would you choose to use in each component of the design?

With mandala art, it is important to experience the creation (or completion through coloring) of a design. Through kinesthetic and nonverbal learning pathways, as is accomplished through coloring, it is possible to deepen one's understanding of these rich and powerful art forms and to get a better feel for how they apply to grand theory structure. Color the mandala in Figure 10.1 with crayons, colored pencils, or paints. Focus on the center and contemplate how the rest of the design symmetrically grows outward. This design has many components; however, the overall effect is one of unity and completeness. While coloring, be mindful of how the components are distinct, yet connected. When the project is complete, close the book and avoid viewing it for several hours or more. When viewed later with a fresh eye, a mandala may appear more unified and hold meanings that were not apparent during the creative process of completing it.

Figure 10.1   Mandala art form. Reprinted with permission from a mandala coloring book created by Monique Mandali. To view more mandalas, or order a mandala coloring book, go to *http://www.mandali.com*.

Learning Activity

Go to the Jones and Bartlett Web site for this text at *http://nursing.jbpub.com* and explore the Web links listed for this chapter.

Myra Estrin Levine's Conservation Model

Myra Estrin Levine (1920–1976) was born in Chicago, Illinois. She was the oldest of three children. Levine developed an interest in nursing because her father was frequently ill and required nursing care on many occasions. Levine graduated from the Cook County School of Nursing in 1944 and obtained her B.S. in nursing from the University of Chicago in 1949. Following graduation, Levine worked as a private duty nurse, as a civilian nurse for the U.S. Army, as a surgical nursing supervisor, and in nursing administration. After earning an M.S. in nursing at Wayne State University in 1962, she taught nursing at many different institutions (George, 2002).

Levine told others that she did not set out to develop a "nursing theory" but had wanted to find a way to teach the major concepts in medical–surgical nursing to undergraduate nursing students over the period of three college quarters. Levine also wished to move away from nursing education practices that were strongly procedurally oriented and refocus on active problem solving and individualized patient care (George, 2002).

The core, or central concept, of Levine's theory is *conservation* (Levine, 1989). When a person is in a state of conservation, it means that individual adaptive responses confront change productively, and with the least expenditure of effort, while preserving optimal function and identity. Conservation is achieved through successful activation of adaptive pathways and behaviors that are appropriate for the wide range of responses required by functioning human beings.

The specific adaptive responses that make conservation possible occur on many levels: molecular, physiologic, emotional, psychologic, and social. These responses are based on three factors (Levine, 1989):

1. *Historicity* refers to the notion that adaptive responses are partially based on personal and genetic past history. Each individual is made up of a combination of personal and genetic history, and adaptive responses are the result of both. In other words, when assessing and supporting adaptive responses in clients, it is necessary for the nurse to take into account both personal and genetic factors when planning care.

2. *Specificity* refers to the fact that each system that makes up a human being has unique stimulus-response pathways. Responses are stimulated by specific stressors and are task oriented. Responses that are stimulated in multiple pathways tend to be synchronized and occur in a cascade of complimentary (or detrimental in some cases) reactions. For example, touching a hot stove will elicit a pain response, an inflammatory response at the site of injury, and an emotional response from the victim, all occurring at about the same time. The pain will cause the victim to rapidly withdraw the hand, resulting in the adaptive response of preventing further tissue damage. The inflammatory response at
   the site of injury will ultimately assist the body to repair and replace damaged tissue. The emotional response will aid the person in remembering what it is like to touch a hot stove so that the mistake will not be repeated in the future.

3. *Redundancy* describes the notion that if one system, or pathway, is unable to ensure adaptation, then another pathway may be able
   to take over and complete the job. This may be helpful when the response is corrective (e.g., the use of allergy shots over a lengthy period of time to diminish the effects of severe allergies by gradually desensitizing the immune system). However, redundancy may be detrimental, such as when previously failed responses are reestablished (e.g., when autoimmune conditions cause a person's own immune system to attack previously healthy tissue in the body).

The product of adaptation is conservation (George, 2002). The nurse's role in conservation is to support patient adaptation and to ensure that the least amount of patient effort is expended to achieve this state. Levine proposes four principles of conservation that should be practiced by nurses, each with unique pathways that are influenced by historicity, specificity, and redundancy. These four principles include (Levine, 1989):

1. The conservation of energy of the individual. (Encourage rest so that the patient has the energy needed for baseline and healing functions.) The conservation of the structural integrity of the individual. (Promote healing with as little further damage, or scarring, to the patient as possible.)
2. The conservation of personal integrity (retaining sense of self) of the individual.
3. The conservation of social integrity of the individual. (Preservation of old, and, when needed, the creation of new connections between patient and social entities outside of self.)

Other assertions, or components, that appear in Levine's work include the following (George, 2002):

- Health and disease are patterns of adaptive change.
- The purpose of nursing is to take care of others when support of adaptive change is needed.
- Optimal health is the goal of conservation.
- The most successful adaptations are those that best support a state of conservation with the least amount of energy expended.
- A person who provides nursing care bears a heavy debt of responsibility when entering into another person's life during vulnerable times when illness has caused temporary dependency.

To summarize, Levine expressed the view that within the nurse–patient relationship a patient's state of health is dependent on the nurse-supported process of adaptation. Effective adaptation leads to conservation, wherein the patient achieves his or her own unique optimal state of health with minimum energy expenditure. The goal of nursing care is to recognize, assist, promote, and support adaptive processes that benefit the patient.

A mandala design representing Levine's Conservation Model might include these components: The central, or focal, point is the concept of conservation. Immediately surrounding this central point are uniform shapes that represent the four principles of conservation. Around each of the four shapes are three identical circles that represent historicity, specificity, and redundancy. Evenly spaced beyond these central concepts are shapes representing supporting concepts that add clarity of meaning to the whole.

Learning Activities

1. To support deeper understanding of Levine's theory, envision and then create a mandala design on page 75. Use the 10 questions listed on page 69 of Chapter 10 as a guide. After completing the mandala, share your creation with your classmates.
2. Find Web sites or journal articles about Levine's theory. Words to use when performing a search might include:
   - Myra Estrin Levine
   - Conservation Model
   - Nursing theory
3. Go to the Jones and Bartlett Web site for this text at *http://nursing.jbpub.com* and explore the Web links listed for this chapter.

Feel free to use these blank pages as a canvas for your learning activities.

Betty Neuman's Systems Model

B etty Neuman was born in Ohio in 1924. She was a middle child with two brothers. When Betty was 11, her father died of kidney disease after several hospitalizations. Betty's father spoke highly of the nurses who cared for him in the hospital, Betty's mother was a rural midwife. Both of these factors played a part in inspiring Neuman to become a bedside nurse.

Neuman could not afford to attend nursing school directly after graduation from high school, so she worked as an aircraft instrument repair technician, draftsperson, and short-order cook while saving for her nursing education and helping to support her mother and younger brother. The creation of the Cadet Nurse Corps Program finally made it possible for Neuman to enter a hospital nursing school. She graduated with a diploma degree from People's Hospital in Akron, Ohio, in 1947. Neuman earned a B.S. in public health nursing in 1957 and an M.S. in public health nursing and mental health nursing from the University of California, Los Angeles, in 1966. In 1985, Neuman was granted a Ph.D. in clinical psychology at Pacific Western University. Neuman also received an honorary doctorate from Grand Valley State in Michigan. Throughout her career as a nurse, Neuman worked in hospital and community health settings in a variety of staff and administrative positions. She also served as nursing faculty, chairing the nursing program from which she graduated. Neuman currently lives and works in Ohio (George, 2002).

The Neuman Systems Model was initially developed in the 1970s for use in nursing education. Neuman sought to create "a unifying focus for a wide range of nursing concerns.... in particular, the model takes into account all variables affecting a client's possible or actual response to stressors and explains how system stability is achieved in relation to environmental stressors imposed on the client" (Neuman & Fawcett, 2002, p. 3).

Neuman's model was influenced by the General Systems Theory, which asserts that the world is made up of connected systems that exert influence on one another. If one system experiences disruption, it will affect all the other associated systems. Larger systems may be made up of layers of smaller systems. Envision a dipped chocolate candy with an inner core of vanilla fluff, then a layer of caramel over the fluff, followed by a layer of nuts over the caramel, then a layer of chocolate over nuts, ending with a layer of coconut over the chocolate. In Neuman's theory, the vanilla fluff would represent the core human being, with the outer layers representing levels of protection for the core.

Neuman's model was also influenced by the General Adaptation Syndrome (Hans Selye, 1907–1982). This syndrome asserts that humans and animals have a nonspecific response to stress that occurs in four stages (Mosby, 1998):

1. *Alarm* occurs when there is an injury or prolonged stress to body or mind.
2. *Resistance* or *adaptation* occurs when various defense mechanisms of the mind and body are mobilized to address the stress.
3. *Exhaustion* results when the mind or body disintegrates.
4. *Adjustment and healing* occur when the mind or body effectively adapts to the stressor.

The General Adaptation Syndrome principles coupled with General Systems Model principles form the basis for the Neuman Systems Model approach of recognizing a structure "that depicts the parts and subparts and their interrelationship for the whole of a client as a complete system." (Neuman & Fawcett, 2002, p. 11). The concepts of *wholism* and *wellness* are discussed in relation to the theory in this way:

The philosophic base of the Neuman Systems Model encompasses wholism, a wellness orientation, client perception and motivation, and a dynamic systems perspective of energy and variable interaction with the environment to mitigate possible harm from internal and external stressors, while caregivers and clients form a partnership relationship to negotiate desired outcome goals for optimal health retention, restoration, and maintenance (Neuman & Fawcett, 2002, p. 12).

Neuman's model recognizes the definitions of the following four concepts that are commonly used in nursing practice: client, environment, health, and nursing (Neuman & Fawcett, 2002):

- The person, family, group, or community are all viewed as a *client* or *client system*. When discussing systems that contain more than one person, boundaries must be clearly defined with regards to who is included in the system and what relationships exist between system members. The client system is a composite of five interacting variables that are in various degrees of development. These variables include physiologic, psychologic, sociocultural, developmental, and spiritual components.
- The *environment* includes all internal and external factors or influences that surround the client or client system.
- The concept of *health* is viewed as a continuum with wellness on one end and illness on the other. Health for the client or client system is equated with optimal system stability, or the best possible state of wellness at any given time.
- The major concern for *nursing* is to keep the client system stable through accurately assessing the effects and possible effects of stressors and assisting with client adjustments to obtain the highest degree of wellness possible at the time.

The following 10 statements summarize the overall approach of the Neuman Systems Model (Neuman & Fawcett, 2002):

1. Each individual client is a unique composite of innate responses that occur within a common range of "normal" as seen within most human beings.
2. The client is in dynamic, constant energy exchange with the environment.
3. Many known, unknown, and universal environmental stressors exist. Each differs in its potential for disturbing a client's usual stability level. Five interrelated variables that make up the client system may affect the degree to which a client is protected from stressors. These five interrelated variables include physiologic, psychologic, sociocultural, developmental, and spiritual aspects of the client system.

4. Each individual has evolved a normal range of responses to the environment that is referred to as the normal line of defense, or usual wellness/stability state. This normal line of defense evolves over time through coping with diverse stressors. The normal line of defense can be used as a standard from which to measure health deviation.

5. A flexible line of defense surrounds and protects the normal line of defense from invasion by stressors. An example of a component that would be a part of this defense would be consistent daily sleep patterns supporting rest, healing, and wellness. This flexible line of defense would be threatened by a change in sleep patterns, such as when a client becomes exhausted due to a lack of regular sleep while working rotating shifts and attending nursing school.

6. The client, whether ill or well, is a dynamic composite of the inter-relationships of physiologic, psychologic, sociocultural, developmen-tal, and spiritual variables. Wellness is determined by the adequacy of energy available to support system stability.

7. Inside each client system, there are internal resistance factors that function to stabilize and return the client to the usual, or possibly an improved, state of wellness following response to a stressor.

8. The nurse may be involved in the process of *primary prevention*, wherein general knowledge is applied in client assessment and preventive healthcare measures aimed at reducing the chance of possible stressors and resultant illness. Health-promotion activities fall within this category.

9. The nurse may be involved in secondary prevention activities, wherein there are symptoms of stress or illness apparent and treatment is pro-vided to decrease the effects of the stressor.

10. The nurse may be involved in tertiary prevention activities, wherein adjustment following illness is supported, and maintenance activities aimed at returning the client system to stability move the client in a circular manner back to primary prevention.

Neuman expressed the view that it is helpful for nurses to approach nurs-ing care using a structured, systems-oriented approach. By doing so, it is pos-sible to discern interrelationships between multiple factors that dynamically influence health and wellness. Stressors cause system instability, and many variables affect a client's ability to regain health and stability after going through a period of stress. Using Neuman's approach, nurses have the opportunity to assess and appropriately address client stressors systematically and thoroughly so that optimal client wellness may be achieved in a variety of situations.

A mandala design representing the Neuman Systems Model might include these components: The central, or focal, point is the concept of a client or client system. The central point is large in the overall scheme of the design. Within the central point are shapes that represent the five interacting variables: physiologic, psychologic, sociocultural, developmental, and spiritual components.

Arranged in concentric circles around the large central point are uniform shapes that represent the four definitions of *client, environment, health,* and *nursing.* Evenly spaced beyond these central concepts are shapes representing the supporting concepts that add clarity of meaning to the whole (Review the 10 summary points on pages 79 and 80).

Learning Activities

1. To support deeper understanding of Neuman's theory, envision and then create a mandala design on page 82. Use the 10 questions listed on page 69 of Chapter 10 as a guide. After completing the mandala, share your creation with your classmates.
2. Find Web sites or journal articles about Neuman's theory. Words to use when performing a search might include:
   - Betty Neuman
   - General Systems Theory
   - General Adaptation Syndrome
   - Neuman Systems Model
3. Go to the Jones and Bartlett Web site for this text at *http://nursing.jbpub.com* and explore the Web links listed for this chapter.

Feel free to use these blank pages as a canvas for your learning activities.

Sister Callista Roy's Adaptation Model

Sister Callista Roy is a member of the Sisters of Saint Joseph of Carondelet. She was born in Los Angeles, California, in 1939. In 1963, Roy earned a B.A. in nursing from Mount Saint Mary's College in Los Angeles and an M.S.N. in 1966 from the University of California, Los Angeles. Roy was awarded an M.A. in sociology in 1973 and a Ph.D. in sociology in 1977, both from the University of California. In the 1980s, Roy served on the faculties of several different institutions.

While completing her M.A., Roy was challenged by one of her nursing teachers, Dorothy E. Johnson, to create a conceptual model for nursing, and that is when she began to develop her Adaptation Model. The Roy Adaptation Model was first published in *Nursing Outlook* in 1970. Since that first journal article in 1970, Roy has published numerous books, chapters, and articles about the Roy Adaptation Model (Tomey & Aligood, 2002). Enthusiastic application and development of this model continue today.

The Roy Adaptation Model applies the two concepts of *systems* and *adaptation* to nursing practice. In the context of Roy's work, the term *system* refers to a grouping of units that are related and connected, thus forming a unified whole. (A system may be an individual, family, group, community, or society.) *Adaptation* refers to effective coping mechanisms that promote integrity for a person, or group of persons, in terms of survival, growth, reproduction, and mastery. In general, Roy asserts that a person is a biophysical being (or system) in constant interaction with a changing environment and that a person has four different modes of adaptation. As internal and external environmental changes occur, needs change that may result in the necessity for active coping to restore integrity. Each client system (either person or group) has a zone that surrounds a variable level of adaptation. Stimuli that fall within the zone of adaptation result in positive adaptations that support integrity. Stimuli that fall outside the zone will result in negative responses that do not support adaptation or integrity (Tomey & Alligood, 2002).

The four modes of adaptation that support integrity are as follows (Roy, 1984):

1. *Physiologic–physical* adaptation for an *individual* occurs when the five needs of oxygen, nutrition, elimination, activity/rest, and protection are met, in addition to adequate neurologic and endocrine function and balanced fluids, electrolytes, and acid-base chemistry. Adaptation for a *group* includes adequate number of participants to achieve goals, shared productive capacities, adequate physical facilities, and fiscal resources.

2. *Self-concept group identity* adaptation for an *individual* occurs when psychic and spiritual integrity promotes a sense of purpose, unity, and meaning in the universe. Adaptation for a *group* includes group identity maintained through honestly shared relations, goals, and values, coupled with a shared sense of achievement.

3. *Role function* adaptation for an *individual* includes knowing who one is in relation to others and involves the use of various adaptive modes suited to the unique multiple roles expected of each individual. Adaptation for a *group* involves enactment of varied role responsibilities that ultimately support the achievement of common goals.

4. *Interdependence* adaptation for an *individual* includes the giving and receiving of love, participating in satisfying relationships, and engaging in meaningful communication. Adaptation for a *group* includes involvement in continually maturing collective relationships and achieving adequate food, shelter, health, and security through interdependence with other group members.

Four major concepts constitute the Roy Adaptation Model:

1. *Humans are wholistic, adaptive systems as both individuals and groups.* "As living systems, persons are in constant interaction with their environments.

Between the system and the environment occurs an exchange of information, matter, and energy. Characteristics of a system include inputs, outputs, controls, and feedback" (George, 2002, p. 298).

2. The *environment* is made up of internal and external stimuli from around the individual or group system. Environment includes "all conditions, circumstances, and influences that surround and affect the development and behavior of humans as adaptive systems, with particular consideration of person and earth resources" (Roy & Andrews, 1999, p. 52).

3. *Health* is defined as "a state and process of being and becoming an integrated whole as a human being.... [*integrity* is defined as] soundness or unimpaired condition leading to wholeness" (Roy & Andrews, 1999, p. 54).

4. The *goal of nursing* is the promotion of the four modes of adaptation, thereby supporting the overall integrity of the human adaptive system. Nurses also seek to reduce ineffective responses through anticipating and addressing potential concerns and also effectively attending to current concerns (George, 2002; Roy & Andrews, 1999).

Roy's Adaptation Model is particularly suited for use with the traditional nursing process. Following is a version of the nursing process as it might be viewed within the context of the Roy Adaptation Model (George, 2002):

- *Assessment of client(s) behavior* involves observing for "actions or reactions under specified circumstances. It can be observable or non-observable" (Roy & Andrews, 1999, p. 67). This activity is consistent with the notion of gathering output from a human system.
- *Assessment of stimuli* involves analyzing patterns of client output to identify ineffective adaptive responses that require nursing intervention.
- *Nursing diagnosis* is created by the nurse and represents an interpretation of how well the human system is adapting to whatever condition or situation brought them to the point of assessment.
- *Goal setting* involves clearly stating the desired outcomes of nursing care, including desired client behavior, specific nature of any expected changes, and the time frame in which this will occur.
- *Interventions* "are planned with the purpose of altering stimuli or strengthening adaptive processes. The nurse plans specific activities to alter the selected stimuli appropriately" (George, 2002, p. 320).
- *Evaluation* assesses the effectiveness of the interventions and involves active input from both the nurse and the client(s). Specifically, "goal behaviors are compared to the client's output responses, and movement toward

or away from goal achievement is determined. If the goals have not been met, then the nursing process begins again.... " (George, 2002, p. 321).

Roy's work has a broad scientific and philosophical foundation that provides the underpinnings of this model. Philosophically, Roy's model supports a "focus on awareness and the notion of eliminating false consciousness, enlightenment to reach self-control, balance, and quietude, and the reclamation of earthly creation as the core of faith" (Roy & Andrews, 1999, p. 35). The following are an additional 10 scientific and philosophical assumptions that influence Roy's Adaptation Model (George, 2002; Roy & Andrews):

1. Systems of matter and energy progress to higher levels of self-organization.
2. Consciousness and meaning demonstrate person–environment integration.
3. Awareness of self and environment is rooted in thinking and feeling, and thinking and feeling mediate human actions.
4. System relationships include acceptance, protection, and fostering of interdependence.
5. Persons and the earth have common patterns and integral relationships.
6. Human consciousness has the power to transform persons and environment.
7. Persons have mutual relationships with the world and God.
8. Human meaning is rooted in an omega-point convergence of the universe.
9. God is revealed in creation.
10. Persons are accountable for the process of transforming the universe.

In summary, the Roy Adaptation Model proposes a structure for nursing practice that focuses on the human being as an adaptive system. This human adaptive system continually interacts with stimuli. On the occasions that a human being, or group of human beings, is unable to maintain wholeness or integrity with respect to necessary life processes, nursing intervention can help to restore adaptation, effective coping, and ultimately optimal health. Nurses work primarily in the realm of supporting adaptive responses, whereas the medical profession focuses more on the health–illness continuum. With conscious collaboration, the two disciplines are able to provide effective client support in times of medical need.

A mandala design representing the Roy Adaptation Model might include these components: The central, or focal, point is the concept of *client/client system*. The central point is large in the overall scheme of the design. Within the central point are shapes that represent the four modes of adaptation: *physiologic/physical, self-concept/group identity, role function,* and *interdependence.* Around the large central point, uniform shapes are intertwined that represent the four major concepts of the model: *client* as adaptive system, *environment* as stimulus, *health* as adaptation/wholistic integrity, and *nursing* as a support to adaptation. In a large circle surrounding these central concepts are shapes that represent each of the steps in the nursing process. Surrounding and enveloping the entire design are shapes representing the supporting scientific and philosophical concepts.

Learning Activities

1. To support deeper understanding of Roy's theory, envision and then create a mandala design on page 90. Use the 10 questions listed on page 69 of Chapter 10 as a guide. After completing the mandala, share your creation with your classmates.
2. Find Web sites or journal articles about Roy's theory. Words to use when performing a search might include:
   - Sister Callista Roy
   - Systems theory
   - Nursing process
   - Adaptation Model
3. Go to the Jones and Bartlett Web site for this text at *http://nursing.jbpub.com* and explore the Web links listed for this chapter.

Feel free to use these blank pages as a canvas for your learning activities.

Dorothea Orem's Self-Care Model

D orothea Orem was born in Baltimore, Maryland, in 1914. Orem earned her diploma in nursing in the 1930s. In 1939, she earned her B.S. in nursing education, which was followed by an M.S. in nursing education in 1945 from the Catholic University of America. She has received many professional awards and honorary degrees. Over her long professional career, Orem has worked as a staff nurse, a private duty nurse, a nursing faculty member, an administrator, and a consultant. Orem's nursing concept of self-care was first published in 1959. She continued to develop this theory and in 1980 published the first edition of *Nursing: Concepts of Practice*, the sixth edition appearing in 2001. Orem continues to develop her theory while working as a nurse consultant.

Orem's Self-Care model is generally stated as follows (Orem, 2001, p. 82):

The condition that validates the existence of a requirement for nursing in an adult is the health-associated absence of the ability to maintain continuously that amount and quality of self-care that is therapeutic in sustaining life and health, in recovering from disease or injury, or in coping with their effects. With children, the condition is the inability of the parent (or guardian) associated with the child's health state to maintain continuously for the child the amount and quality of care that is therapeutic.

Orem's Self-Care Model is composed of the three interrelated concepts of self-care, self-care deficit, and nursing systems (George, 2002).

Self-care involves the four aspects of self-care, self-care agency, basic conditioning factors, and therapeutic self-care demand. *Self-care* is what people plan and do on their own behalf to maintain life, health, and well-being. When self-care is effectively performed, it helps maintain structural integrity and human functioning and contributes to human development (George, 2002; Orem, 2001). *Self-care agency* is a person's acquired ability to engage in self-care. Self-care agency is affected by *basic conditioning factors* that include age, gender, developmental and health state, sociocultural factors, healthcare system factors, family system factors, patterns of living, environmental factors, and adequacy/availability of resources. *Therapeutic self-care demand* refers to what is needed at various times in a person's life when health care is required to meet self-care needs through the use of appropriate actions and interventions (George, 2002). Orem identifies the following primary needs that must be met by human beings to ensure adequate self-care (George, 2002; Orem, 2001):

1. Sufficient intake of air, water, and food
2. Adequate care and functioning of elimination
3. Balance between activity and rest
4. Balance between solitude and social interaction
5. Prevention of hazards to human life, functioning, and well-being
6. Promotion of functioning and appropriate development within social groups in accord with human potential, limitations, and the human desire to be normal

When a person is in the position of needing medical care to diagnose and/or correct an illness, adequate self-care also includes the following (Orem, 2001):

1. Seeking and securing medical help when needed
2. Responsibly attending to the effects and results of pathologic conditions
3. Effectively carrying out prescribed interventions
4. Responsibly attending to the regulation of effects resulting from prescribed interventions
5. Accepting the fact that sometimes self or others need medical help when faced with certain life challenges
6. Learning to live productively with the effects of pathologic conditions and treatments while promoting continued personal development

Self-care deficit results when adults or parents with dependent children are incapable of providing continuously effective self-care. Nursing care may be required if there is a need for education to enhance self-care abilities, if there is a current deficit in self-care abilities, or if it is anticipated that self-care abilities will decrease in the future. The five methods of helping, to be used alone or in combination when there is concern over a self-care deficit, are (Orem, 2001):

1. Acting for or doing for another
2. Guiding and directing
3. Providing physical or psychological support
4. Providing and maintaining an environment that supports personal development
5. Teaching

Nursing systems are designed by nurses based on an assessment of the individual's self-care needs. "If there is a deficit between what the individual can do (self-care agency) and what needs to be done to maintain optimum functioning (therapeutic self-care demand), then nursing is required" (George, 2002, p. 131). Orem has described three kinds of nursing systems that are meant to meet the variable needs of individual situations. These three systems include (George, 2002):

1. The *wholly compensatory system* is one in which patient action is limited and the nurse accomplishes most of what is required to maintain therapeutic self-care, compensates for the patient's inability to engage in self-care, and supports and protects the patient.
2. The *partially compensatory system* is one in which the patient and nurse work together to meet self-care requirements, with the patient performing some of the tasks necessary for successful self-care and the nurse performing whatever else is required.
3. The *supportive-educative system* is one in which the patient provides necessary self-care, and the nurse and patient work together to regulate the exercise and development of self-care agency.

These three combined concepts of self-care, self-care deficit, and nursing systems make up a general Self-Care Model with a three-step nursing process that can be compared with the widely used *nursing process*. Orem's three steps follow, with corresponding nursing process steps provided in parentheses (George, 2002):

1. Diagnosis and prescription includes determining why nursing care is needed through careful analysis and interpretation of information gathered while assessing the patient. This is the step when nurses make professional judgments regarding what care to provide (assessment and nursing diagnosis, including desired outcomes).
2. Design of a nursing system and plan for delivery of care to achieve desired outcomes (plans with scientific rationale).
3. Production and management of nursing systems (implementation and evaluation).

In summary, Orem's Self-Care Model describes a structure wherein the nurse assists the client, where needed, to maintain an adequate level of self-care. The degree of nursing care and intervention depends on the degree to which the client is able (or unable) to meet self-care needs. This theory is structured in such a way that the concepts are straightforward to understand and apply. The simplicity of wording, coupled with an uncanny resonance with everyday nursing activities, has ensured its broad popularity and use in many areas of nursing.

A mandala design representing Orem's model might contain these components: There is a large central point divided into three lobes representing *self-care*, *self-care deficit*, and *nursing systems*. Streaming outward from the self-care lobe is a shape that encompasses the four concepts of self-care, self-care agency, basic conditioning factors, and therapeutic self-care demand. Streaming outward from the self-care deficit lobe is a shape that encompasses the five methods of helping. Streaming outward from the nursing systems lobe is a shape that encompasses the three systems of nursing care. Encircling the periphery of the design are Orem's three nursing process steps.

Learning Activities

1. To support deeper understanding of Orem's theory, envision and then create a mandala design on page 98. Use the 10 questions listed on page 69 of Chapter 10 as a guide. After completing the mandala, share your creation with your classmates.

2. Find Web sites or journal articles about Orem's theory. Words to use when performing a search might include:
   - Dorothy Orem
   - Self-Care Model
3. Go to the Jones and Bartlett Web site for this text at *http://nursing.jbpub.com* and explore the Web links listed for this chapter.

Feel free to use these blank pages as a canvas for your learning activities.

Madeleine Leininger's Culture Care: Diversity and Universality Theory

Madeleine Leininger was born in Sutton, Nebraska. In 1948, she received her diploma in nursing from St. Anthony's School of Nursing in Denver, Colorado. In 1950, she earned a B.S. from St. Scholastica (Benedictine College) in Atchison, Kansas, and in 1954 earned an M.S. in psychiatric and mental health nursing from the Catholic University of America in Washington, D.C. In 1965, she was awarded a Ph.D. in cultural and social anthropology from the University of Washington, Seattle (Tomey & Alligood, 2002).

Early in her career as a nurse, Leininger recognized the importance of the concept of "caring" in nursing. Frequent statements of appreciation from patients for care received prompted Leininger to focus on "care" as being a central component of nursing. During the 1950s, while working in a child guidance home, Leininger experienced what she describes as a cultural shock when she realized that recurrent behavioral patterns in children appeared to have a cultural basis. Leininger identified a lack of cultural and care knowledge as the missing link to nursing's understanding of the many variations required in patient care to support compliance, healing, and wellness (George, 2002). These insights were the beginnings (in the 1950s) of a new construct and phenomenon related to nursing care called *transcultural nursing*.

Leininger is the founder of the transcultural nursing movement in education research and practice. In 1995, Leininger defined transcultural nursing as:

> a substantive area of study and practice focused on comparative cultural care (caring) values, beliefs, and practices of individuals or groups of similar or different cultures with the goal of providing culture-specific and universal nursing care practices in promoting health or well-being or to help people to face unfavorable human conditions, illness, or death in culturally meaningful ways (p. 58).

The practice of transcultural nursing addresses the cultural dynamics that influence the nurse–client relationship. Because of its focus on this specific aspect of nursing, a theory was needed to study and explain outcomes of this type of care. Leininger creatively developed the Theory of Culture Care: Diversity and Universality with the goal to provide culturally congruent wholistic care.

Some scholars might place this theory in the middle range classification. Leininger holds that it is not a grand theory because it has particular dimensions to assess for a total picture. It is a wholistic and comprehensive approach, which has led to broader nursing practice applications than is traditionally expected with a middle-range, reductionist approach. (Personal communication with Penny Glynn on September 12, 2003).

Leininger's theory is to provide care measures that are in harmony with an individual or group's cultural beliefs, practices, and values. In the 1960's she coined the term *culturally congruent care*, which is the primary goal of transcultural nursing practice. Culturally congruent care is possible when the following occurs within the nurse-client relationship (Leininger, 1981):

> Together the nurse and the client creatively design a new or different care lifestyle for the health or well-being of the client. This mode requires the use of both generic and professional knowledge and ways to fit such diverse ideas into nursing care actions and goals. Care knowledge and skill are often repatterned for the best interest of the clients...Thus all care modalities require *coparticipation of the nurse and clients (consumers) working together* to identify, plan, implement, and evaluate each caring mode for culturally congruent nursing care. These modes can stimulate nurses to design nursing actions and decisions using new knowledge and culturally based ways to provide meaningful and satisfying wholistic care to individuals, groups or institutions (Leininger, 1991, p. 44).

Leininger developed new terms for the basic tenets of her theory. These definitions and the tenets are important to understand. Understanding such key terms is crucial to understanding the theory. Below is a basic summary of the tenets that are essential to understand with Leininger's theory (summarized from Leininger, 2001, pp. 46–47):

- *Care* is to assist others with real or anticipated needs in an effort to improve a human condition of concern or to face death.
- *Caring* is an action or activity directed toward providing *care*.
- *Culture* refers to learned, shared, and transmitted values, beliefs, norms, and lifeways of a specific individual or group that guide their thinking, decisions, actions, and patterned ways of living.
- *Cultural care* refers to multiple aspects of *culture* that influence and enable a person or group to improve their human condition or to deal with illness or death.
- *Cultural care diversity* refers to the differences in meanings, values, or acceptable modes of care within or between different groups of people.
- *Cultural care universality* refers to common *care* or similar meanings that are evident among many cultures.
- *Nursing* is a learned profession with a disciplined focused on care phenomena.
- *Worldview* refers to the way people tend to look at the world or universe in creating a personal view of what life is about.
- *Cultural and social structure dimensions* include factors related to religion, social structure, political/legal concerns, economics, educational patterns, the use of technologies, cultural values, and ethnohistory that influence cultural responses of human beings within a cultural context.
- *Health* refers to a state of well-being that is culturally defined and valued by a designated culture.
- *Cultural care preservation or maintenance* refers to nursing care activities that help people of particular cultures to retain and use core cultural care values related to healthcare concerns or conditions.
- *Cultural care accommodation or negotiation* refers to creative nursing actions that help people of a particular culture adapt to or negotiate with others in the healthcare community in an effort to attain the shared goal of an optimal health outcome for client(s) of a designated culture.
- *Cultural care repatterning or restructuring* refers to therapeutic actions taken by culturally competent nurse(s) or family. These actions enable or assist a client to modify personal health behaviors toward beneficial outcomes while respecting the client's cultural values.

There are several specific assumptions inherent in this theory that support the theory premises and Leininger's use of the terms described above. These assumptions are the philosophical basis of Culture Care: Diversity and Universality theory. They add meaning, depth, and clarity to the overall focus to arrive at culturally competent nursing care. The following are distilled from Leininger's work and preceeded other nurses' use in recent years who are now valuing and using these ideas and the theory. These statements are derived from Leininger's key sources (Leininger 1978, 1981, 1991, 1995, 2002, but most specifically, 2001, pp. 44–45):

- Care is the essence and central focus of nursing.
- Caring is essential for health and well-being, healing, growth, survival, and also for facing illness or death.
- Culture care is a broad wholistic perspective to guide nursing care practices.
- Nursing's central purpose is to serve human beings in health, illness, and if dying.
- There can be no curing without the giving and receiving of care.
- Culture care concepts have both different and similar aspects among all cultures of the world.
- Every human culture has folk remedies, professional knowledge, and professional care practices that vary. The nurse must identify and address these factors consciously with each client in order to provide wholistic and culturally congruent care.
- Cultural care values, beliefs, and practices are influenced by worldview and language, as well as religious, spiritual, social, political, educational, economic, technological, ethnohistorical, and environmental factors.
- Beneficial, healthy, satisfying culturally based nursing care enhances the well-being of clients.
- Culturally beneficial nursing care can occur only when cultural care values, expressions, or patterns are known and used appropriately and knowingly by the nurse providing care.
- Clients who experience nursing care that fails to be reasonably congruent with the client's cultural beliefs and values will show signs of stress, cultural conflict, noncompliance, and ethical moral concerns.

In synthesizing the information contained in the defining terms and assumptions just presented, a broad definition emerges of a culturally competent nurse who:

- Consciously addresses the fact that culture affects nurse–client exchanges
- With compassion and clarity, asks each client what their cultural practices and preferences are
- Incorporates the client's personal, social, environmental, and cultural needs/beliefs into the plan of care wherever possible
- Respects and appreciates cultural diversity, and strives to increase knowledge and sensitivity associated with this essential nursing concern.

In summary, nurses who understand and value the practice of culturally competent care are able to effect positive changes in healthcare practices for clients of designated cultures. Sharing a cultural identity requires a knowledge of transcultural nursing concepts and principles, along with an awareness of current research findings. Culturally competent nursing care can occur only when client beliefs and values are thoughtfully and skillfully incorporated into nursing care plans. Caring is the core of nursing. Culturally competent nursing guides the nurse to provide optimal wholistic, culturally based care. These practices also help the client to care for himself and others within a familiar, supportive, and meaningful cultural context. Continual improvement and expansion of modern technologies and other nursing and general science knowledge are integrated into practice if they are appropriate. Today nurses are faced daily with unprecedented cultural diversity because of the increasing number of immigrants and refugees. Commitment to learning and practicing culturally competent care offers great satisfaction and many other rewards to those who can provide wholistic supportive care to all patients (Leininger 1991, 2002).

A mandala design representing Leininger's model might be viewed as a mandala of the primary colors arranged in overlapping circles. The places where the colors overlap create new colors; for example, the place where blue and red overlap creates the color purple. The primary colors represent cohesive cultures that intermingle with others in a limited way, thereby maintaining a strong group identity. The mixed colors represent different cultures that are influenced by multiple cultures. All of the interwoven colors represent many cultures interacting to varying degrees and forming functional communities in an ever-widening circle of interaction and inclusion. The shapes in the design would have symmetry and balance to suggest unity and harmony among them.

Learning Activities

1. To support deeper understanding of Leininger's theory, envision and then create a mandala design on page 107. Use the 10 questions listed on page 69 of Chapter 10 as a guide.
2. Share the mandala you created with classmates.
3. Find Web sites about Leininger's Theory, or search for journal articles. Words to use when performing a search might include:
   - Madeleine Leininger
   - Cultural care
   - Diversity
   - Transcultural Nursing Care
4. Go to the Jones and Bartlett Web site for this text at *http://nursing.jbpub.com* and explore the Web links listed for this chapter.

Feel free to use these blank pages as a canvas for your learning activities.

Theories About Specific Nursing Actions, Processes, or Concepts: Middle-Range Theories

PART

IV

Envisioning Theories Through Origami Art

Theories about specific nursing actions, processes, or concepts (*middle-range theories*) seek to define and provide direction for specific nursing activities. Middle-range theories are those in which nursing topics are most readily identifiable, and nurses who wish to follow the actions or steps described in a theory may do so. Nurses also may be able to replicate or simulate the experience described in the theory. For example, a middle-range theory might propose that there are six steps to productive mentoring relationships between experienced nurses and new nurses. Using the theory as a guide, it would be relatively straightforward for a nurse manager to institute and evaluate the effectiveness of using this six-step approach for mentoring new hires in her unit. If the approach turns out to be effective, then the nurse manager has implemented a valuable tool to enhance consistency of training for new hires. If the approach turns out to be less than helpful, then knowledge has been gained regarding applicability of the theory in this setting. Information has also been provided about mentoring techniques that may not be helpful within this nurse manager's particular pool of staff nurses. With either outcome, useful knowledge has been generated that will clarify for the staff nurses and the manager which approach might be most useful when mentoring new hires.

Envision origami when exploring theories that seek to describe a specific nursing action or process (middle-range theory). Origami is the art of following specific steps for folding paper into recognizable designs or forms (see Color Plates 16.1 and 16.2 in the color insert). The word *origami* is Japanese; however, people in all cultures have engaged in paper folding since the invention of mass-produced paper roughly a century ago. In the United States, many children experiment with the process of folding paper into readily identifiable objects such as party hats, sailboats, and paper airplanes.

The art of origami consists of steps or actions that are meant to lead to a specific outcome or result, and likewise, middle-range theories consist of steps or actions that are meant to lead to a specific outcome or result. In nursing, the steps lead to a readily identifiable outcome related to care, and in origami the steps lead to a readily identifiable concrete object. In either case, carefully planned steps and actions are meant to lead to a concrete, desired outcome.

To create origami, one begins with a flat, square piece of paper that does not resemble a recognizable object. With careful step-by-step folding, the paper becomes something recognizable, such as an animal, flower, insect, boat, or airplane. The idea is simple: Decide what object will be evident after the folding is complete, such as an airplane, and then carefully fold the paper over and over again, until the airplane is done. If a friend folds a particularly good airplane, the best way to figure out how to make one just like it is to carefully unfold the creation and then follow the folds (or steps) to re-create it, learning how to replicate the design. Nursing research based on middle-range theories follows this same process of choosing a desired outcome and then following the steps provided in the theory to hopefully recreate the desired result.

Using a piece of copy paper or wrapping paper, create the origami airplane as shown in Figure 16.1.

The steps involved in the exploration of middle-range theories are similar to the steps involved in producing origami. The following are steps to use when exploring middle-range theories; the corresponding origami steps are in italics:

1. Identify what the concrete outcome of interest is, for example, effective mentoring. *Identify what object will be produced, for example, a sailboat.*

Origami Art

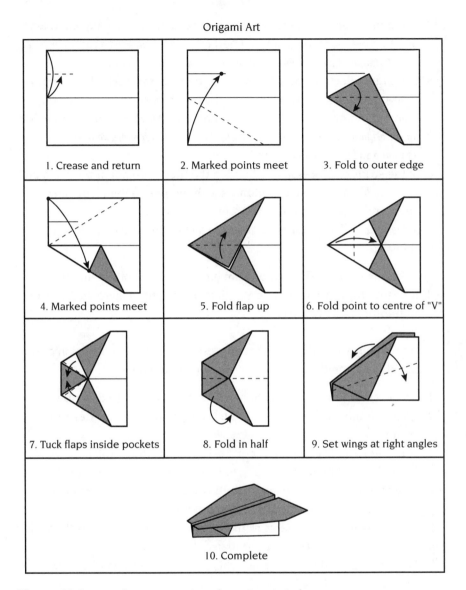

Figure 16.1 Step-by-step creation of an origami airplane.

This traditional origami model airplane was downloaded on May 25, 2003, from Dave's Origami Emporium, *http://members.aol.com/ukpetd/*

2. Determine what processes or steps, for example, those meant to lead to effective mentoring, are outlined in the theory. *Find a pattern or series of fold sequences for transforming a sheet of paper into a sailboat.*

3. Through reflection and personal experience, assess whether the process or series of steps outlined in the theory resonate with personal understanding of effective nurse mentoring. *After completing all of the folds in the origami pattern, assess how closely the creation resembles your understanding of what a sailboat should look like.*

4. If the steps or processes outlined in the theory do not appear to match personal/professional experiences with the phenomenon of nurse mentoring, then explore a different theory or create a new one. *If the completed creation does not look like a sailboat, try another pattern or create a new one.*

Try creating some traditional origami art. Be mindful of the importance of each fold (or step) in completing the finished object. Figure 16.2 presents another traditional pattern to try.

When reading about theories that address a specific nursing action or process (a middle-range theory), ask yourself these questions:

1. What is the purpose of this theory? What is it meant to describe?
2. What are the steps outlined by the theory to achieve the desired result?
3. Are there a sufficient number of steps, and are they explained well enough that others would be able to replicate the desired result?
4. Does the overall pattern and resulting object, or process, resonate with personal/professional nursing experience?
5. What nursing environments would be appropriate to use this theory in?
6. Where would it *not be appropriate* to use the theory?
7. Would it be productive to share this theory with others who work in environments where it might fit?

Learning Activity

Go to the Jones and Bartlett Web site for this text at *http://nursing.jbpub.com* and explore the Web links listed for this chapter.

Origami Art

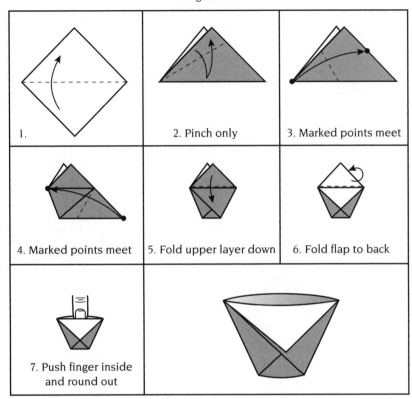

Figure 16.2   Origami drinking cup.

This traditional origami drinking cup was downloaded on May 25, 2003, from Dave's Origami Emporium, *http://members.aol.com/ukpetd/*

Ida Jean Orlando-Pelletier's Nursing Process Theory

I da Jean Orlando-Pelletier was born August 12, 1926, to Italian immigrants. She grew up during the Depression and received a diploma in nursing in 1947 from New York Medical College, Flower Fifth Avenue Hospital School of Nursing. She earned a B.S. in public health nursing in 1951 from St. John's University in Brooklyn, New York. In 1954, Orlando-Pelletier earned her M.A. in mental health consultation from Columbia University Teachers College. During her years of educational progression, Orlando-Pelletier worked in a variety of nursing settings. After completing her M.A., Orlando-Pelletier taught for 8 years at the Yale School of Nursing in New Haven, Connecticut. While at Yale, Orlando-Pelletier was a research associate and principal investigator of a federal project grant entitled "Integration of Mental Health Concepts in a Basic Curriculum," during which time she collected data while observing students interact with patients and other members of the educational and healthcare team. After analyzing these data, Orlando-Pelletier reported her findings in a book published in 1961 entitled *The Dynamic Nurse–Patient Relationship: Function, Process, and Principles of Professional Nursing Practice* (1990). Since its initial publication, the book has been published in five other languages in addition to English. The information in this book forms the foundation of Orlando-Pelletier Nursing Process theory (Tomey & Alligood, 2002).

Orlando-Pelletier Nursing Process theory is based on the premise that the nurse–patient relationship is reciprocal, meaning that the actions of one affect the other. Orlando-Pelletier is one of the first nursing leaders to recognize the pivotal importance of patient participation and intelligent nurse deliberation in the nursing process. Orlando-Pelletier also believes that the nursing profession is distinct from the medical profession and that "nursing action is derived from the patient's immediate experience and immediate needs for help" (Tomey & Alligood, 2002, p. 400). Said another way, Orlando-Pelletier's theory asserts that "nursing is unique and independent because it concerns itself with an individual's need for help, real or potential, in an immediate situation. The process by which nursing resolves this helplessness is interactive and is pursued in a disciplined manner that requires training. She [Orlando-Pelletier] believes one's actions should be based on rationale, not protocols" (George, 2002, p. 191). Orlando-Pelletier's work is considered to be a middle-range theory because it proposes a specific process of deliberative, intentional one-to-one interaction between the nurse and patient to support optimal nursing care directed at addressing a patient's expressed need for help.

The basis of Orlando-Pelletier's Nursing Process theory consists of the three concepts of *patient behavior, nurse reaction that is explored with the patient,* and *nurse action* (George, 2002).

1. "The nursing process is set in motion by *patient behavior.* All patient behavior, no matter how insignificant, must be considered an expression of a need for help until its meaning to a particular patient in the immediate situation is understood.... Patient behavior may be verbal or nonverbal" (George, 2002, p. 193). Verbal behavior encompasses a patient's use of language and nonverbal behavior includes physiological symptoms, motor activity, and nonverbal communication. When a patient has a need for help that cannot be resolved without the help of another, helplessness results. If a patient's behavior does not effectively communicate an accurate depiction of the need for help, then difficulties in the nurse–patient relationship may arise and make it difficult for the nurse to adequately care for the patient. Resolution, or a clearer understanding of ineffective patient behavior, becomes a high priority for the nurse because the situation will likely worsen over time and make adequate care, or the provision of needed help, increasingly difficult. The nurse's actions and reactions are designed to

resolve ineffective patient behaviors and also meet immediate needs for patient help (George, 2002).

2. Patient behavior stimulates a *nurse reaction*, which is the start of the nursing process (Orlando, 1972). Appropriate nurse reaction consists of the following steps (George, 2002):
   - The nurse perceives the behavior through any of the senses.
   - The perception leads to an automatic thought.
   - The thought produces an automatic feeling.
   - The nurse shares reactions with the patient to ascertain whether perceptions are accurate or inaccurate.
   - The nurse consciously deliberates about personal reactions and patient input in order to produce professional deliberative actions based on mindful assessment rather than automatic reactions.

3. A nurse may act in one of two ways when providing care: automatic or deliberative. Professional *nursing actions* are nursing-care activities that result from deliberative activity on the part of the nurse, rather than automatic reactions. Behaviors that stem from automatic rather than deliberative reactions do not meet the criteria for professional nursing behavior. Automatic reactions stem from nursing behaviors that are performed to satisfy a directive other than the patient's need for help. For example, the nurse who gives a sleeping pill to a patient every evening because it is ordered by the physician, without first discussing the need for the medication with the patient, is engaging in *automatic, nondeliberative* behavior. This is because the reason for giving the pill has more to do with following medical orders (automatically) than with the patient's immediate expressed need for help (George, 2002). The criteria for deliberative actions are as follows (George, 2002):
   - Deliberative actions result from the correct identification of patient needs by validation of the nurse's reaction to patient behavior.
   - The nurse explores the meaning of the action with the patient and its relevance to meeting his need.
   - The nurse validates the action's effectiveness immediately after completing it.
   - The nurse is free of stimuli unrelated to the patient's need [when action is taken].

It can be argued that all nursing actions are meant to help the client and should be considered deliberative. However, for an action to have been truly deliberative, it must undergo reflective evaluation to determine if the action helped the client by addressing a need as determined by the nurse and client in the immediate situation (George, 2002).

Assumptions that are inherent in Orlando-Pelletier's approach include the following (Tomey & Alligood, 2002):

- Nursing is allied with medicine and is also a distinct profession separate from other healthcare disciplines.
- Professional (deliberative) nursing has a distinct outcome product from other professions.
- The nurse's mind is the major helping tool.
- Each nurse–patient interaction is unique.
- The nurse's practice is improved by self-reflection.
- The nurse–patient interaction constitutes a dynamic whole.
- The actual nurse–patient encounter is a major source of nursing knowledge.
- Evidence of relieving distress is determined by the client's observable behavior.
- Promptly addressing a patient's need for help is important because the length of time a patient's needs go unmet influences the degree of distress.

Orlando (1990) aptly summarizes her theory as follows:

A deliberative nursing process has elements of continuous reflection as the nurse tries to understand the meaning to the patient of the behavior she observes and what he needs from her in order to be helped. Responses comprising this process are stimulated by the nurse's unfolding awareness of the particulars of the individual situation (p. 67).

An origami design to express Orlando-Pelletier's Nursing Process theory would be a simple design with three large folds representing the three steps, or processes, of *patient behavior, nurse reaction,* and *nurse action.* Subsequent smaller folds would include the assumptions associated with the theory. The finished object might resemble a silhouette of two people connected to one another, alluding to the ongoing nurse and client interaction required for deliberative care to effectively take place.

Learning Activities

1. Perform an Internet search, using the word *origami*, to view galleries of completed origami art. Choose one visual representation that depicts Orlando-Pelletier's theory, print a copy of it, and paste it onto page 122. Underneath the picture, write a few sentences about why this particular origami creation depicts Orlando-Pelletier's theory. Share your picture with your classmates.

2. In relation to Orlando-Pelletier's theory, answer the seven questions found on page 114.

3. Find Web sites or journal articles on Orlando-Pelletier's theory. Words to use when performing a search might include:
   - Ida Jean Orlando-Pelletier
   - Nursing process
   - Nursing Process theory

4. Go to the Jones and Bartlett Web site for this text at *http://nursing.jbpub.com* and explore the Web links listed for this chapter.

Feel free to use these blank pages as a canvas for your learning activities.

Katharine Kolcaba's Theory of Comfort

Katharine Kolcaba was born December 28, 1944, in Cleveland, Ohio. She received a diploma in nursing from St. Luke's Hospital School of Nursing in Cleveland. She then practiced for many years as a medical-surgical nurse, a long-term care nurse, and a homecare nurse. In 1987, Kolcaba graduated in the first R.N. to M.S.N. class at Case Western Reserve University. While completing her master's degree, Kolcaba worked in a dementia unit, and it was there that she began theorizing about the concept of comfort. Upon completion of her M.S.N. degree, Kolcaba became a faculty member at the University of Akron College of Nursing. Kolcaba received a Ph.D. in nursing in 1997 from Case Western Reserve and is certified in gerontology (Tomey & Alligood, 2002). She continues to teach and has published numerous articles discussing the concept of comfort as it relates to nursing. She has also published a book entitled *Comfort Theory and Practice: A Vision for Holistic Health Care and Research* (2003).

Kolcaba's Theory of Comfort specifically addresses the practice concept of nurse-provided comfort. It also describes a process by which comfort may be consistently delivered and evaluated by nurses. For these reasons, it is considered to be a middle-range theory.

Kolcaba's theory is based on the premise that one of most important nursing activities is that of providing comfort. The function of nursing, according to Kolcaba, is (Tomey & Alligood, 2002)

> ....the intentional assessment of comfort needs, design of comfort measures to address those needs, and reassessment of comfort levels after implementation compared to the previous baseline. Assessment and reassessment may be intuitive and/or subjective, such as when a nurse asks if the patient is comfortable, or objective, such as in observations of wound healing, changing lab values, or changes in behavior. Assessment can be achieved through the administration of visual analogue scales or traditional questionnaires.... (p. 434).

The recipients of care may include individuals, family groups, institutions, or communities.

In a general sense, the term *comfort* could be defined as the experience of receiving effective care that meets comfort needs. There are three types of comfort and four contexts within which comfort occurs (Kolcaba, 1994). The three *types of comfort* defined by Kolcaba (1996) include the following:

1. *Relief* is the state of a patient who has had a specific need met.
2. *Ease* is a state of overall calm and contentment.
3. *Transcendence* is a state in which a person rises above problems and pain.

The experience of comfort occurs within different contexts. A desired result of appropriate comfort care would be optimal functioning in the following four contexts (Kolcaba, 1996):

1. *Physical* pertains to bodily sensations and homeostatic mechanisms.
2. *Psychospiritual* pertains to internal awareness of self, including esteem, sexuality, and life's meaning. It also includes a person's relationship to a higher being.
3. *Environmental* pertains to external surroundings, conditions, and influences. The environment may be altered by the patient, nurse, or others to enhance comfort.
4. *Sociocultural* pertains to interpersonal, family, and societal relationships, as well as family traditions, rituals, and religious practices.

Nurses provide comfort through *comfort measures* that are designed to meet the needs of individual patients. Comfort needs may be associated with physical, psychospiritual, environmental, or sociocultural factors (Kolcaba,

1994). Comfort needs are expressed by the patient and assessed by the nurse through nurse monitoring of verbal or nonverbal reports, pathophysiologic parameters, education deficits, need for support, and financial stresses. *Intervening variables*, which are factors that influence a patient's perception of total comfort, might include past experiences, age, attitude, emotional state, support system, prognosis, and finances. The specific combinations of the number and types of *comfort measures needed, context,* and *intervening variables* influence a patient's overall perception of the level and type of comfort experienced.

Four broad assumptions and theoretical assertions that help form the basis of Kolcaba's work are listed here. Knowledge of these assumptions clarifies the meaning of the theory (Kolcaba, 1994):

- Human beings have wholistic responses to complex stimuli.
- Comfort is a wholistic outcome of effective nursing care.
- Human beings have a need for comfort and will seek comfort wherever possible.
- Nurses are in a position to identify the comfort needs of their patients, design comfort measures, and assess outcomes to support enhanced comfort.

In summary, the presence or absence of patient comfort is an often-addressed issue in nursing practice. Kolcaba's Theory of Comfort lends structure and meaning to the term *comfort* as it applies to the nurse–patient relationship. Kolcaba (1994) stated, "The understanding of comfort directly guides nursing care that is inclusive of physical, psychospiritual, social and environmental interventions.... Clinicians have the capability and disciplinary interest to effect comfort, and patients look to nurses for help in achieving comfort" (p. 1183). Exploration and explanation of this often-used concept will allow nurses to formally study the phenomenon of comfort and discern care practices that will support optimal patient comfort.

An origami design that might express Kolcaba's Theory of Comfort would consist of seven folds representing the three levels of comfort (*relief, ease,* and *transcendence*), and the four contexts in which comfort occurs (*physical, psychospiritual, environmental,* and *sociocultural*). The finished object would resemble a patchwork quilt, representing the *comfort* one might experience when wrapped up in a warm, handmade quilt on a rainy day.

Reflections About Comfort Theory

Kathy Kolcaba

Some of you know that I wrote *Comfort Theory* (CT) because it was required for my dissertation. Specifically, a theory was required to underpin my mandatory comfort study and thus required for graduation. My dilemma was that there were no nursing theories that remotely referred to patient comfort, so I looked at earlier nursing dissertations for any existing theory that would have the following criteria: it had to have a high level of abstraction (so I could link comfort into it), it had to be centered on patients (because ideas were related to their comfort needs), and it had to have adequate explanatory power (so I could learn something from it). Lo and behold, I found Edward Murray's framework from the 1930s, recently used by a graduate of our program, and I was able to link comfort and other nursing concepts beneath his original generic ones. My lower theoretical level was more concrete and specific to health care than Murray's, and I called that level my mid-range theory of comfort. I was able to place comfort, which needed a home, right at the heart of it all.

My newly formulated theory served nicely for my dissertation study, but when I told my advisor I wanted to try to publish it before my dissertation was completed (another 2–3 years), she balked. She didn't want me to take the time to do this—but I did it anyway, quietly, and CT was published about a year later. This style of being a theorist became the norm for me, in that my ideas did not come out of thin air; they were initiated by external forces beyond my control, they were controlled by institutional politics, and they were not given enthusiastic support at first. I did not let myself be deterred when my theoretical work was rejected for conference presentations. Even though I did not yet have data to support CT, I stubbornly believed that this idea of comfort should be central to nursing much as it was at the beginning of our profession. Indeed, perhaps comfort is needed even more in modern nursing, as an antidote to all the high-tech equipment. Also, my zodiac sign is Capricorn, and I always thought that the goat was a good description of how I plodded along toward my goal of broad acceptance of CT, going around or over hurdles by finding greener pastures *somewhere*, all the while making modest headway by putting one foot in front of the other.

Another important factor for me was that, as a teacher, I had the discretion of imposing CT on my own students and observing what worked and didn't work for them and their patients. What I saw was that the students enjoyed intentionally comforting their patients in many technical and not-so-technical ways and (yes …) including all of these ways on their daily comfort care plans. Unlike the usual sterile nursing process format, comfort care plans required that students record everything they did for their patients, including such comforting interventions as repositioning, rubbing patients' backs, walking and talking with them, cleaning up their rooms, etc. Because comfort care plans are holistic, students could record their interventions in no particular order after they identified individual comfort needs, and they could record their patients' responses to these interventions. This sort of documentation then provided a very complete and unique picture of each patient. Of course, the patients loved all this attention to their comfort, too. And together, through positive and negative feedback from students and patients, CT became richer, more relevant, and more useful. For example, students questioned me about the lack of emphasis on physiological problems in CT, so I saw that I needed to strengthen my definition of physical comfort. They asked, "Who cares about patient comfort besides the patient?" and I added the concept of institutional integrity to the model. For the advancement of CT, this sort of feedback was and is invaluable to me. So valuable, in fact, that I continue to teach my theory course in the summer, even though I am otherwise retired from the University of Akron after teaching full time for 22 years.

While waiting for my wannabe presentations to be more widely heard, my theory to be published in nursing textbooks, and nursing politics to discover that comfort is an outcome that patients and families want and need, I was adding students' ideas and observations about patients who were comforted to my Web site. Because updating could occur quickly on the Web, this became my preferred venue for modifying CT and for building my network with like-minded students and nurses. Come visit me in cyberspace at www.ThecomfortLine.com.

When Magnet status was created to reward nurse-friendly hospitals, I saw an opportunity to take my theory on the road. The Magnet award gave a big boost to nursing theory in general because the criteria for Magnet were many, expensive, and difficult to achieve, requiring that all nurses and administrators in a given hospital be on the same page. This was much easier if nurses utilized a theory for focus. CT was particularly pertinent because nurses could use it to improve their working environment, so I redefined the four contexts of comfort in terms of nurses' comfort. Nurses loved being asked, first by me and then by their bosses, for their comfort wish lists—ideas that would turn their workplaces into comfort zones.

I never intended to be an entrepreneur, but I began my business called *The Comfort Line* (named after my Web site) as a way to promote nursing, specifically the *art* of nursing in which nurses comfort their patients and families in many creative, satisfying ways. Even though most nurses were doing this intuitively, modern charting provided no place to report comfort work, and so it was undervalued by administrators and underrecognized by the general public.

Therefore, when introducing CT to a new class or audience, I often ask for personal experiences if they or a family member had been recipients of nursing that made a difference. Their stories (I call them "memorable nurse" stories) show how meaningful those nursing acts of compassion and comforting are for healing. Usually, nurses who comforted them were the only ones the students remembered.

Why was comfort important for healing? The original meaning of comfort, or *confortare*, is "to strengthen greatly." I refer to this meaning frequently to propose that patients who are comforted do better in surgical healing, therapies, and learning new regimens for health and discharge planning (health-seeking behaviors). This made administrators interested, because their financial bottom line (or institutional integrity) could be improved. With nurse leaders, I also suggested that institutions that adopted CT for their practice framework would find that their nurses would be more productive (remember the comfort wish lists), better able to comfort and strengthen their patients, and more likely to stay in that hospital system because their work was satisfying and visible.

Recently, patient satisfaction became an important national and public measuring stick for how hospitals compare with others. So I again adapted CT to this trend. In this way, I found that, if I kept on top of the trends, I could adapt CT to fit most innovations or needs in health care today. I could also instantly adapt the material on my Web site and make it and myself available through new and nifty technologies that students and many practicing nurses would value, such as podcasts and webcasts. Getting patient comfort accepted politically remains my most difficult challenge—gatekeepers at the highest levels of nursing are frustratingly inaccessible and/or closed to ideas outside their boxes.

I had many lucky stars that lined up to guide my way and support me when I got tired or discouraged. These stars include my graduate programs and professors at Case Western Reserve University, my students at the University of Akron, my family, my research team members, nurses in my consulting hospitals, and the patients and families who demonstrated the significance of comforting interventions in ways large and profound. All of these stars enabled this old goat to plod along toward the next adaptation and application of CT. (Actually, at this writing, I am a very spry and adventuresome 64 years.) I hope that you will all consider being future guiding lights for comfort theory. Thank you, one and all!

Learning Activities

1. Perform an Internet search using the word *origami* to view galleries of completed origami art. Choose one visual representation that depicts Kolcaba's theory, print a copy of it, and paste it onto page 132. Underneath the picture, write a few sentences about how this particular origami creation depicts Kolcaba's theory. Share the project with classmates.
2. In relation to Kolcaba's theory, answer the seven questions found on page 114.
3. Find Web sites or journal articles about Kolcaba's theory. Words to use when performing a search might include:
    *   Katharine Kolcaba
    *   Comfort
    *   Comfort care
    *   Theory of comfort care
4. Go to the Jones and Bartlett Web site for this text at *http://nursing.jbpub.com* and explore the Web links listed for this chapter.

Feel free to use these blank pages as a canvas for your learning activities.

Nola Pender's Health-Promotion Model

N ola Pender was born in Lansing, Michigan, in 1941. She was an only child, and her parents were advocates for the education of women. At the age of 7, Pender took note of the nursing care her hospitalized aunt received, and this prompted an early interest in nursing. Further education strengthened her interest in obtaining a nursing degree, and with family support, Pender received her diploma from the School of Nursing at West Suburban Hospital in Oak Park, Illinois, in 1962. She then worked in medical-surgical and pediatric nursing. She completed a B.S.N. at Michigan State University in East Lansing in 1964. In 1965, Pender earned an M.A. in human growth and development from Michigan State University and in 1969 completed a Ph.D. in psychology and education at Northwestern University in Evanston, Illinois. Several years after completing her Ph.D., Pender completed master's level studies in community health nursing at Rush University in Chicago. Since 1990, Pender has been professor and associate dean for research at the University of Michigan School of Nursing. Pender has published many articles about exercise, behavior change, and relaxation training and has edited many journals and books. The fifth edition of her book on her Health Promotion Model was published in 2006.

Pender (2003) explains the importance of health promotion as follows:

Very early in my nursing career, it became apparent to me that health professionals intervened only after people developed acute or chronic disease and experienced compromised lives. Attention was devoted to treating them after the fact. This reactive approach did not reflect the philosophical beliefs of our predecessors in nursing who focused on maintaining conditions of a healthy interaction between self and the environment.... I committed myself to the proactive stance of health promotion and disease prevention with the conviction that it is much better to experience exuberant well-being and prevent disease than let disease happen when it is avoidable and then try and cope with it.

Health-promoting behaviors are a desired outcome when providing client care and education. Health-promoting behaviors may be defined as an action directed toward attaining positive health outcomes such as optimal well-being, personal fulfillment, and productive living (Tomey & Alligood, 2002). Examples of health-promoting behaviors include eating a healthy diet, exercising regularly, managing stress, gaining adequate rest, enhancing spiritual growth, and building positive relationships. Nurses in all practice areas have numerous opportunities to encourage health-promoting behaviors related to presenting concerns and anticipated health challenges. Pender (1996) identifies the following factors as having a potential influence on the health-promoting behaviors of clients. Whereas the first two items on the list (prior related behavior and personal factors) are difficult (or impossible) for a nurse to change, the other factors listed can be influenced positively by nurses through effective assessment, support, and education. Pender's (1996) factors include the following:

- *Prior related behavior* refers to the past frequency of behaviors. The more frequently a behavior was done in the past, the more likely it is that the behavior will continue in the future.
- *Personal factors* include biological, psychological, and sociocultural factors that directly and indirectly influence health-promoting behaviors.
  - *Biological factors* include age, gender, body mass index, onset of puberty or menopause, aerobic capacity, strength, agility, and balance.
  - *Psychological factors* include self-esteem, self-motivation, personal competence, perceived health status, and individual definition of health.
  - *Sociocultural factors* include race, ethnicity, cultural identity within the larger culture, educational opportunities, and socioeconomic status.
- *Perceived benefits of action* are the expected positive outcomes of the proposed health-promoting behavior. For example, a teenager may

be prompted to quit smoking after the nurse comments that smoking causes teeth to become discolored and that after quitting teeth will remain whiter and healthier.

- *Perceived barriers to action* are the real and imagined barriers to health behavior change. For example, financial limitations might make it impossible for a client to maintain a membership at a gym (a real barrier). Another client may be able to pay for the gym membership only to be thwarted by an imagined barrier such as, "Everyone will laugh and stare at me every time I go to the gym because I am not in good physical condition."
- *Perceived self-efficacy* refers to personal judgment about individual capability to organize and consistently perform new behaviors. Higher self-efficacy results in lowered perceptions of possible barriers to positive health behavior change. For example, if a person perceives himself or herself as being well organized and motivated toward self-betterment, that person is less likely to encounter significant barriers to behavioral change than someone who feels disorganized and unmotivated.
- *Activity-related effect* refers to negative and positive behaviors associated with actually doing the health-promoting behavior. For example, if a person resolves to walk a mile during lunch break every day at work and finds that the result is fatigue and unpleasantly sweaty work clothes, then the feelings associated with the actual activity of walking for fitness at work may be negative.
- *Interpersonal influences* refer to how the significant others around the client affect motivation for positive change. These influences include expectations, social support, and modeling by family, peers, and healthcare providers. If a client lives in a household where all the adults smoke, then smoking cessation will be more difficult than if the client is the only adult who smokes and the rest of the family would prefer for them to quit.
- *Situational influences* refer to external factors that affect the client's perception of the proposed health-promoting behavior, such as where, when, and how the activity will take place. For example, if a client is asked to attend a nutritional education class in the lobby of a candy store, the smell and inviting appearance of the candy might make it impossible for the client to commit to a weight loss program unless the competing demand of the irresistible candy is removed.

- *Commitment to a plan of action* refers to the person's intention to change and the creation of a plan of action to accomplish the implementation of a health-promoting behavior. Clients are more likely to engage in health-promoting behaviors when they anticipate realizing specific benefits from the activity.
- *Immediate competing demands* are behaviors over which the client has little control because they are associated with necessary life activities, such as work or family care responsibilities. For example, if a client had to choose between leaving a child home alone to go to the gym or staying home with the child, most parents would choose to stay home rather than leave the child alone. In this situation, exploring exercise options that would include time spent with the child may be more effective in the long run than attempting to complete an exercise regime at a gym.
- *Competing preferences* are those choices over which a client has a high degree of control, such as whether to eat an apple or a candy bar for an afternoon snack. Education regarding healthy rather than poor food choices would enable the client to adjust personal preferences and make better-informed decisions that would support healthy eating behaviors.

Knowledge of the assumptions that form the foundation of a theory are helpful in clarifying the overall thrust and meaning of the theory. Pender's Health Promotion Model is based on the following assumptions (Pender, 2003; Pender, Murdaugh, & Parsons, 2002):

- Individuals seek to create conditions of living through which they can express their unique human potential.
- Individuals have the capacity for reflective self-awareness, including assessment of their own competencies.
- Individuals value growth in directions viewed as positive and attempt to achieve a personally acceptable balance between change and stability.
- Individuals seek to actively regulate their own behavior.
- Individuals in all their biopsychosocial complexity interact with the environment, progressively transforming the environment and themselves over time.
- Health professionals constitute a part of the interpersonal environment, which exerts influence on persons throughout their life span.
- Self-initiated reconfiguration of person–environment interactive patterns is essential to behavior change.

Many nurse theorists create diagrams or abstract visual representations of theory concepts. Most of these creations require comprehensive knowledge and understanding of a theory before they can be fully appreciated or understood. Because Pender's model is relatively simple and self-explanatory, it is included here (see Figure 19.1).

In summary, Pender's Health Promotion Model proposes a structured process for assessing and addressing client needs associated with healthy behaviors. This model is based on combined nursing and behavioral health approaches that are meant to help clients make positive health behavioral

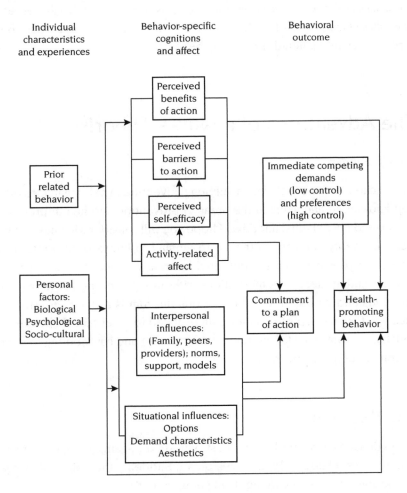

Figure 19.1   Pender's Health Promotion Model. Pender, N. (2005). *Health Promotion in Nursing Practice* (5th ed.). Upper Saddle River, NJ: Prentice Hall.

changes. Pender's model provides immediately applicable principles to help nurses systematically address this important issue. Nurses who are aware of specific concerns related to promoting healthy behavior are more effective in supporting long-term positive health behaviors and activities for all clients.

An origami design to express Pender's Health Promotion Model might be a simple design depicting an apple (remember the old saying, "An apple a day keeps the doctor away"?). The first two folds of the design would represent *prior related behavior* and *personal factors*. Subsequent folds would incorporate the factors that nurses are able to assist clients in changing, such as *perceived benefits, perceived barriers, self-efficacy, activity-related effect, interpersonal influences, situational influences*, and *immediate competing demands*. The last fold would represent a *commitment to a plan of action*. The final result of all of these folds would be an apple representing health-promoting behaviors.

The Adventures of a Nurse Theorist

Nola J. Pender

I am excited to share with you my lifelong adventure in helping nurses develop knowledge and skills in the areas of prevention and health promotion. As you read my personal narrative, I hope you will consider what new insights, ideas, or theory you can contribute to nursing to improve our profession. I know that every nurse has the potential for creative work because I hear endless fascinating ideas in conversations with nurses. Getting our ideas out of our heads and on paper for others to benefit from is a challenge. However, once you take a deep breath and plunge ahead to meet that challenge, your work has the potential for altering nursing forever and contributing to the development of our beloved profession.

The Beginning

A man thrashes in his bed as his chest pain strikes again. He looks at me with anxious eyes. Please help, his eyes plead. Suddenly the pain strikes again, and he cries, "I am going to die! I am going to die!"

A woman who is diabetic and markedly overweight is trying to work out at the fitness center at the hospital. She looks at me, perspiring profusely and trying to get her breath. "I just can't do this, I just can't do this," she gasps. "Why did I ever let myself get in this shape?"

A small child looks up at me with sad eyes. She was playing with matches at home and her clothes caught on fire. She knows that today her bandages will need to be changed and she is gripped with fear.

These are the images that I encountered as I worked as a nurse in medical-surgical and pediatric settings. I began to wonder why nurses could not *prevent* such tragic human situations. All this suffering might have been prevented with healthy lifestyles and healthy environments.

As I pursued my graduate education, I began to read about wellness. Halbert Dunn wrote about high-level wellness. John Travis wrote about a wellness life-style. I asked myself, was high-level wellness wishful thinking or was it really attainable? Then I had that aha moment—helping people achieve the highest level of health or wellness possible to maximize quality of life is what nursing is all about. Wellness is the goal of nursing as Florence Nightingale intended it to be. Wellness and health promotion needed much more attention in nursing!

Family members play a crucial role in the direction our life takes. In my case, my husband, who had just completed his doctorate, urged me to go on for doctoral work. His support was crucial in the next phase of my life as a budding theorist. I pursued a doctoral degree at Northwestern University with a dual major in education and psychology. The more immersed I became in learning about how people think and make decisions, the more motivated I became to combine nursing and psychology to create a model to help nurses understand how people can change their thinking and behavior to adopt healthy lifestyles. I was excited, motivated, and having fun trying to organize my thoughts about critical aspects of health counseling by nurses.

Along the Way

After I finished by doctoral degree, I accepted my first teaching position at Northern Illinois University. After I taught for 3 years, we had our first child, a daughter. The next year we had our son. Two wonderful children! As I looked into their eyes, I was even more motivated to move nursing in the direction of health promotion. If we could create healthy lifestyles for children by working with them and their families, then healthy living would unfold early in life and hopefully carry forward into adulthood. Being a mother was a continuing source of motivation to make a difference in nursing, for the sake of my children and thousands of children worldwide.

People are our inspiration at each step in life. I had very special colleagues at Northern Illinois University. Dr. Beverly McElmurry inspired me with her interest in health as the focus for nursing curricula. Drs. Susan Walker, Karen Sechrist, and Marilyn Stromborg and I began discussions about the role of nurses in promoting healthy living. By that time, I had drafted a health promotion model (HPM) that combined ideas from nursing, education, and psychology about the trigger points for promoting health behavior change. My colleagues and I decided to apply for research monies to test the model and see if it worked. We were funded for a total of 5 years of research to test the HPM with adults. The model did predict health behaviors, but after looking at the research findings carefully, we decided that a model that had behavior-specific variables might be even more predictive and helpful. Thus, after our discussion, the health promotion model was revised. For example, rather than focusing on self-esteem, we adopted Dr. Albert Bandura's concept of self-efficacy or confidence in ability to perform a specific behavior. Other changes were made also. A model or theory evolves as research findings indicate how to improve it. Ideas that spring from our heads or that we adapt from another field are just that—ideas—they need to be tested; that is what we accomplish through our research.

After I moved to the University of Michigan, further funding for research allowed me to test the HPM with children and physical activity. The model did have some predictive power, which was encouraging. Other colleagues at the University of Michigan were also testing the model. Dr. Sally Lusk and her colleagues developed an extensive research program testing the HPM with adults in regard to hearing protection and conservation. It was encouraging to see that an intervention based on the HPM did increase worker use of hearing protection.

The next adventure in testing the HPM was a funded pilot study conducted with Dr. Lorraine Robbins and Dr. Kimberlee Gretebeck to test a nurse practitioner counseling intervention to increase physical activity among middle school girls. With this pilot intervention, we saw changes in beliefs, but we did not see significant changes in physical activity. That was a disappointment. However, not easily discouraged, we went back to the drawing board to see what we could do to increase the impact of the intervention. Currently, Dr. Robbins is funded to test the enhanced intervention with adolescent girls from diverse cultures. The results of her study will determine if the behavioral counseling intervention for adolescent girls, based on the HPM, really does improve their level of physical activity.

In addition to the aforementioned studies, many other research studies, including dissertations, have been conducted using the HPM. It is fun to get e-mails almost every day from students asking for further information about the model or telling me about their work with the model.

Looking Ahead

I am very fortunate to have made a contribution to nurses' awareness of the importance of health promotion and to their knowledge and ability to counsel patients for lifestyle change. However, theories and models are not created in a vacuum. Many people motivate and inspire us along the way. Our patients, our families, our coworkers, and the writings of professionals who have gone before us all fuel our interest, our thoughts, and our passion for creative work in nursing. In my case, the spark for a lifelong career came from seeing patients in distress whose distress might have been prevented through healthy living. Your spark may be another life-changing clinical experience.

As the science for evidence-based practice continues to evolve, the profession of nursing needs new models and theories. New theories that are better than older ones emerge, and the new theories replace theories from the past. That is the natural evolution of knowledge in nursing. By being alert to your clinical environment, listening to your patients and colleagues, and playing with clinical ideas in new combinations, you, too, can become a nurse theorist. We need your contribution to nursing, both now and for the future. Remember, for theories to be of value to nursing, they must be useful. They must help us with our everyday interactions with patients. Theories or models that begin in nursing interactions and nursing observations are most likely to serve nursing well as we continue to develop as a caring science. Join the adventure!

Learning Activities

1. Perform an Internet search using the word origami to view galleries of completed origami art. Choose one visual representation that depicts Pender's model, print a copy of it, and paste it onto page 145. Underneath the picture, write a few sentences about how this particular origami creation depicts Pender's model. Share your picture with your classmates.
2. In relation to Pender's model, answer the seven questions found on page 114.
3. Find Web sites or journal articles about Pender's model. Words to use when performing a search might include:
   - Nola Pender
   - Health promotion
   - Health promotion model
4. Go to the Jones and Bartlett Web site for this text at *http://nursing.jbpub.com* and explore the Web links listed for this chapter.

Feel free to use these blank pages as a canvas for your learning activities.

Hildegard Peplau's Interpersonal Relations in Nursing

H ildegard Peplau was born in Reading, Pennsylvania, in 1909. In 1931, Peplau graduated from the Pennsylvania School of Nursing and began her nursing career. She earned a B.A. in interpersonal psychology from Bennington College, Vermont. Peplau also completed an M.A. in psychiatric nursing in 1947 and an Ed.D. in curriculum in development in 1953 at Teachers College in Columbia, New York. Peplau taught graduate psychiatric nursing at Columbia University, New York, then taught at Rutgers University for 20 years, earning the title of "Professor Emeritus." Peplau died peacefully in Sherman Oaks, California, in 1999.

During her long career, Peplau contributed greatly to the development of psychiatric nursing and to the advancement of nursing as a profession. In 1952, Peplau's book, *Interpersonal Relations in Nursing*, described the relationship between nurse and client. Peplau is considered a visionary because she published this work during a time when the creation of nursing theories was not a focal point in the profession (George, 2002). Many believe that this book caused a shift in perception from the accepted practice of the nurse performing interventions *on or to* a patient to the nurse and patient acting in partnership during the care process (Tomey & Alligood, 2002).

Peplau (1988) broadly describes nursing as:

a significant, therapeutic, interpersonal process. It functions co-operatively with other human processes that make health possible for individuals in communities .... Nursing is an educative instrument, a maturing force that aims to promote forward movement of personality in the direction of creative, constructive, productive, personal, and community living (p. 16).

Understanding and applying Peplau's theory first requires participant observations by the nurse in three focal areas. The nurse must consciously observe:

1. His or her own behaviors
2. The behaviors demonstrated by the patient
3. The type and quality of relations that occur between nurse and patient

This calls for honest, and sometimes uncomfortable, self-appraisal by the nurse that is meant to ultimately result in the nurse becoming more aware of what messages are being communicated to the patient (Peplau, 1997). Gaining a better understanding will help the nurse avoid interpersonal pitfalls within the nurse–patient exchange, such as (Peplau, 1997):

- Labeling the patient, either intentionally or unintentionally
- Comparing the patient with others
- Competing with the patient by trying to "one-up" them in some way
- Taking advantage of the patient by using care time to talk about the nurse's personal experiences rather than the patient's
- Expecting the patient to change after one nurse–patient interaction
- Declining to discuss difficult or emotional topics with the patient
- Avoiding patients rather than honestly addressing anger or annoyance

Peplau describes multiple roles that the nurse may fulfill within a nurse–patient relationship. These roles are best managed if the nurse actively observes and appraises self, patient, and the quality of relations on an ongoing basis. Some of the roles include (Peplau, 1952, 1988):

- Stranger
- Teacher
- Healthcare resource person
- Leader
- Counselor

- Safety agent
- Mediator
- Observer

The nurse may fulfill many roles in addition to those just listed when providing care to individuals. Enactment of a role should depend on the need of the patient at any given time. Through careful observation, nurses are able to choose what role might fit best within specific situations to support optimal patient outcomes.

Three overlapping phases representing the structure of nurse–patient relationship have been described by Peplau (1997):

1. The *orientation phase* is when the nurse and patient are getting acquainted with one another. This is when the nurse clarifies what she or he will do within the nurse–patient relationship. It is also when the nurse gains information on what the patient wants and expects from the relationship. Active listening on the part of the nurse is especially important during this phase (although listening is important in all phases).
2. The *working phase* is when most of the pointed and intense interaction occurs and is also when the nurse is likely to assume multiple roles in the relationship as needed in order to help the patient experience a positive outcome. Through self-evaluation and careful observation, nurses may professionally mature during the working phase through increasing understanding of how and why they relate to individual patients in certain ways.
3. The *termination phase* is when nurses and patients summarize the work accomplished and move toward closure of the relationship. Discharge planning is usually initiated prior to starting the termination phase so that patients have an opportunity to gradually move toward termination rather than experience an abrupt transition at the end of care.

In summary, *Peplau's Interpersonal Relations in Nursing* describes a basic framework within which nurses and patients interact. Because it describes one component of nursing care (the interaction between patient and nurse), it is a middle-range theory. However, the basic nature of this theory allows for its application by every nurse in a wide range of situations. This theory is profoundly important because it was the first to propose that instead of *doing things to* a patient, a nurse must *provide care in partnership with* the patient.

An origami design to express Peplau's Interpersonal Relations in Nursing theory might be a design consisting of three different colors of paper: one representing the patient, one representing the nurse, and one representing the relationship. The three papers are intertwined into the form of a triangle with three sides, each side made up of all three colors. The completed triangle represents the completed relationship, consisting of the three sides, or steps, of the relationship: the orientation phase, the working phase, and the termination phase. The symmetry and form of the design symbolize the positive and satisfying interpersonal exchange that results for both the nurse and the patient when the nurse consciously employs the concepts described by Peplau.

Learning Activities

1. Perform an Internet search, using the word *origami* to view galleries of completed origami art. Choose one visual representation that depicts Peplau's model, print a copy of it, and paste it onto page 151. Underneath the picture, write a few sentences about how this particular origami creation depicts Peplau's model. Share your project with your classmates.
2. In relation to Peplau's model, answer the seven questions on page 114.
3. Find Web sites or journal articles on Peplau's theory. Words to use when performing a search might include:
   - Hildegard Peplau
   - Interpersonal Relations in Nursing
4. Go to the Jones and Bartlett Web site for this text at *http://nursing.jbpub.com* and explore the Web links listed for this chapter.

Feel free to use these blank pages as a canvas for your learning activities.

Imogene King— Conceptual System and Theory of Goal Attainment

I mogene M. King, who developed the theory of goal attainment, was born on January 30, 1923, in West Point, Iowa. King earned a diploma in nursing from St. John's Hospital School of Nursing in St. Louis, Missouri, in 1945, and a bachelor's and master's of science degree in nursing from St. Louis University in 1948 and 1957, respectively. King worked as an instructor and assistant director at the St. John's Hospital School of Nursing from 1947 until 1958 while working on her bachelor's and master's degrees. King studied under Mildred Montag, creator of associate degree nursing at Teachers College, Columbia University, earning her Ed.D. in 1961 (Messmer, 2009).

After receiving her doctoral degree, Dr. King worked as an associate professor of nursing at Loyola University, where she began publishing her work on nursing theory (Tomey & Alligood, 2006). King served as the Assistant Chief, Research Grants Branch, Division of Nursing, in Washington, DC, from 1966 to 1968 under Dr. Jessie M. Scott. From 1968 to 1972, King was director and professor in the school of nursing at Ohio State University. Her book, *Toward a Theory for Nursing: General Concepts of Human Behavior* (1971), was published during her tenure at Ohio State. In 1972, King returned to Loyola University, where she coordinated clinical research in the School of Nursing until 1980, when she moved to the University of South Florida in Tampa as a professor of nursing. She worked at South Florida until her retirement in 1990. After her retirement, she continued to work with the King International Nursing Group (KING) to advance her theory. King, a Sigma Theta Tau International Virginia Henderson fellow, was a recipient of the Elizabeth Russell Belford Founders Award for Excellence in Education. In 1994, she was inducted into the American Academy of Nursing and in 1996, received the Jessie M. Scott Award from the American Nurses Association.

King enjoyed eclectic interests, including abstract painting, golf, politics, and daytime soap operas (Messmer, 2009). King gave generously of her time to help students better understand her theory, allowing her e-mail address to be published on Eichelberger's Nursing Theory Web site. She communicated daily with students and others interested in her theory. However, she was adamant that a Web site on her theory not be created. Members of KING were working on a KING Web site, when King asked that they stop. She appeared to be uncomfortable with the Web and concerned that her work would be misrepresented (Bev Whelan, personal communication, April 20, 2008). She never married and died at the age of 84 on Christmas Eve, 2007, in Florida. King's papers and memorabilia are at Loyola University in Chicago, Illinois.

Conceptual System

In 1971, King wrote her first textbook, which outlined a conceptual framework, later called a conceptual system, which nurses could use to identify and analyze nursing situations. King's framework was a "way of thinking about the real world of nursing" (King, 1971, p. 125). She also outlined the process of developing theory as either inductive or deductive, where one could develop a theory and then test it in practice through research or develop theory deduced from research data. King stated that both methods had value.

King's work is considered a conceptual model by some because it encompasses both a conceptual framework and a theory (Fawcett, 2000). King's conceptual view of nursing is based on Von Bertanlanffy's general systems theory, which influenced her to study the complexity of nursing by identifying and analyzing the interdependent variables and concepts that exist in phenomena (King, 2007). King defined a system as a set of components linked by communication that exhibit directed behaviors for the purpose of attaining goals, thus giving rise to her theory of goal attainment (King, 1997).

In King's view, the goal of nursing is to assist individuals to attain, maintain, or restore their health. To achieve this outcome, nurses and clients engage in interactions of verbal and nonverbal communication where information is exchanged and interpreted. The outcome of this process is a transaction where values, needs, and wants are shared. King views this interactive process between client and nurse as the essential element of nursing. King (1996) explained the relationship between the four major nursing metaparadigms (humans, nursing, health, and environment) by stating that the domain of nursing involves human beings, families, and communities in a framework where nurses conduct transactions in various environments with the goal of attaining, maintaining, or restoring health.

King wrote that all people grow and develop within nations, which, in turn, make up societies throughout the world, giving a sense of global community. This commonality depicts the communication and interaction that occurs within small groups in their nations' social networks. Three changing and interactive systems, the personal, interpersonal, and social systems, make up most societies throughout the world, according to King (2006).

Assumptions

The assumptions within King's model are many, and for a more complete listing, please refer to King's original sources or Fawcett's chapter on King (Fawcett, 2005; King, 1981, 1997). King's model and theory of goal attainment are based on her overarching belief that the focus of nursing is people interacting with their environment, which leads to a state of health and the ability to function in social roles (King, 1981). A basic assumption of King's goal attainment theory is that the nurse and client communicate information, set mutual goals, and then act to attain those goals. Factors that affect the attainment of goal are roles, stress, space, and time.

Major assumptions related to the four metaparadigms of nursing are as follows:

Human Beings/Persons:

- are open, social beings who are unique, rational, sentient, and capable of making decisions.
- have the ability to perceive, think, feel, choose, and set goals and select means to achieve goals.
- have values that are linked to their culture and dictate their behavior and goals.
- differ in their needs, desires, and goals.
- have three fundamental needs, which include the following:
  - health information
  - care that seeks to prevent illness
  - care when they are unable to help themselves

Health:

- is the dynamic life experiences of a human being, which calls for the continuous adjustment to stressors in the internal and external environment causing the optimum use of one's resources to achieve maximum potential for daily living.
- is a changing state where variations are constant and ongoing.
- is made up of genetic, subjective, relative, dynamic, environmental, functional, cultural, and perceptual characteristics (King, 1990).

Environment

- Environment is the background for human interactions.
- Environment involves internal and external components where
  - internal environment transforms energy to enable humans to adjust to continuous external changes.
  - external environment involves formal and informal organizations and is a source of stress and continuous changes.
- Understanding the ways in which humans interact with their environment to maintain health is necessary for nursing professionals (King, 1981).

Nursing

- Nursing is a goal-seeking system where the performance of roles and responsibilities assist human beings to attain, maintain, and restore health (King, 1971).
- Nursing is a series of actions, reactions, and interactions where the nurse and client exchange information and perceptions and set goals and determine the means to achieve the goals.
- Human beings and their actions are the focus of nursing.
- Perceptions of the nurse and the client influence the interaction process (King, 1981, p. 143).

Concepts

King's conceptual model identifies the domain of nursing as a composite of the following three major interacting systems: personal systems (individuals), interpersonal systems (groups), and social systems (society). These three systems provided the basis for King's theory of goal attainment. Humans are the basic element in each of the systems and the unit of analysis is human behavior in various social environments. King identified 15 concepts and placed them within one of the three systems. However, King readily admits that the concepts are not limited to one system but rather cut across all of the systems.

Personal System

Personal systems are made up of individuals and include the client and nurse functioning as a total system. An individual is described as "a unified being, or self, who perceives, thinks, desires, imagines, decides, and identifies goals to be achieved" (King, 1981, p. 19). A personal system includes seven dimensions, which include perception, self, growth and development, time, body image, learning, and personal space (Fawcett, 2005).

In the personal system, King views the concept of perception as the process of organizing, interpreting, and transforming information from sensory data and memory. Perception is part of the process of human transactions with the environment. Perception gives meaning to one's experience, represents one's image of reality, and influences one's behavior (King, 1981, p. 24). King considered perception to be the most important element within the personal system because of its influence on behavior. One's "perceptions of self, of body image, of time and space influence the way he or she responds to persons, objects, and events in his or her life" (King, 1981, p. 19).

The concept of self is seen as the human being's inner world. Self is who a person perceives himself to be. Growth and development refer to the continuous changes that occur inside and outside of human beings. Growth and development, according to King, include all changes that occur even at the cellular level and are influenced by genetics, lived experiences, and the environment (King, 1981).

Time is the duration between events and is unique to each person. The perception of time is subjective and an irreversible succession of events. Body image is "an individual's perceptions of his/her own body, others' reactions to his/her appearance which results from others' reaction to self" (King, 1981, p. 33). A person's body image is influenced by others' reaction to him or her and the person's interactions with others.

Learning is a "process of sensory perception, conceptualization, and critical thinking involving multiple experiences in which changes in concepts, skills, symbols, habits, and values can be evaluated in observable behaviors and inferred from behavioral manifestations (King, 1986, p. 24). Personal space is the immediate environment in which nurse and client interact and move toward goal attainment (King, 1981, p. 149). Space exists in all directions and the physical area or territory communicates role, position, and interactions with others. Space is situational, dimensional, transactional, and dependent of the perception of the person (King, 1981).

Interpersonal System

Interpersonal systems consist of groups or individuals interacting with one another. King refers to two individuals interacting as dyads, three individuals as triads, and four or more individuals as small or large groups (1981). The more individuals who are involved, the more complex the system becomes.

The concepts associated with interpersonal systems are interaction, transaction, communication, role, coping, and stress.

Interactions are the acts of two or more people who are in contact with each other. Interactions occur in concrete situations where human beings are actively participating and moving toward the achievement of a goal. Interactions can reveal how individuals feel about other humans, what expectations exist, and how each reacts to the actions of the other. A transaction is the process of interacting where humans communicate with others and the environment for the purpose of achieving goals that they value. Transactions are goal-directed human behaviors (King, 1981, p. 82). Interactions and transactions between nurse and client constitute an interpersonal system.

Communication is the processing of information where a change occurs from one state to another. According to King, communication is the sharing of thoughts, perceptions, and opinions among individuals using verbal and nonverbal messages to create social interaction and learning opportunities (1981).

Roles are considered a set of behaviors expected from someone who is occupying a certain position in a social framework. Roles are occupied by one or more individuals interacting in a specific setting for a specified purpose. Coping is viewed as a person's ability to handle stressors. Knowledge of coping is necessary for the interpersonal system.

Stress is an energy response of a person to specific people, objects, and/ or events that can be perceived as positive or negative stressors. Stress is a "dynamic state whereby a human being interacts with the environment to maintain balance for growth, development, and performance which involves an exchange of energy and information between the person and the environment for regulation and control of stressors" (King, 1981, p. 98).

Social System

The third interacting system is the social system. Social systems are groups of people within a community or society who share common goals, interests, and values. A social system has organized boundaries including roles, behaviors, and practices. A social system can be a family, school, or coworkers. The concepts identified within the social systems are organization, authority, power, status, control, and decision making.

An organization can be viewed as a system whose activities are oriented toward the achievement of goals. An organization is made up of a group of human beings with assigned roles and positions who use resources and abilities to accomplish personal and organization goals. Authority is a "transactional process characterized by active, reciprocal relations in which members' values, backgrounds, and perceptions play a role in defining, validating, and accepting the directions of individuals within an organization" (King, 1981, p. 124). Authority is the power to make decisions directing the actions of human beings. Authority may lie in the position one holds or the level of expertise, skill, or depth of knowledge a person possesses.

Power is the ability to use resources to achieve goals. Power is having influence over others in situations. Power defines a situation in a way that people will accept what is being done whether they agree with it or not. Power is situational (King, 1981, p. 127).

Status is the position of a person or a group relative to other groups in an organization. Status is related to who you are, what you do, who you know, and what you have achieved (King, 1981, p. 130). Control is a dimension of the concept of the social system (King, 1986). Decision making is a "dynamic and systematic process by which a goal-directed choice of perceived alternatives is made, and acted upon by individuals or groups to answer a question and attain a goal" (King, 1981, p. 132).

Summary

The relationships between the three systems—personal, interpersonal, and social systems—make up King's theory of goal attainment. The conceptual framework of the interpersonal system had the greatest influence on the development of this theory. King (1981) stated, "Although personal systems and social systems influence quality of care, the major elements in a theory of goal attainment are discovered in the interpersonal systems in which two people, who are usually strangers, come together in a health care organization to help and to be helped to maintain a state of health that permits functioning in roles" (p. 142). King believed that interactions between the nurse and the client lead to transactions that result in goal attainment and enhanced growth and development of clients.

Nurses have set goals for their patients most likely from the beginning of professional nursing. However, King examined the process of setting goals from a nursing theory perspective and developed a conceptual framework for nursing, out of which arose a usable nursing theory.

King's theory has been used by nurses working in a variety of settings with many different patient populations. While King's theory has been criticized for its vague explanation of environment (Fawcett, 2005) and its inability to be applied to clients who cannot participate in their care (Tomey & Alligood, 2006), nurses have and continue to use King's system and theory to implement theory-based practice.

Learning Activities

1. Recall a client you have cared for recently and briefly list the issues your client had related to each of the dimensions in King's personal system—perception, self, growth and development, time, body image, learning, and personal space.
2. King believed that the interpersonal systems had the greatest influence on a client's quality of care. Do you agree or disagree? Explain your position.
3. Identify the most compelling part of King's theory of goal attainment. Briefly describe the component and explain why you feel this is the most interesting part of King's theory.

Web Sites

www.kingnursing.org

> King International Nursing Group (KING)—KING was established in the 1990s to foster the development of nursing knowledge based on the work of Dr. Imogene King. It was deactivated for a period of time but was reactivated in August 2009 to honor her work.

http://library.loyno.edu/services_collections/streaming/?id=33

> Streaming video of King's interview—Helene Fuld Foundation Portraits of Excellence

Patricia Benner— Model of Skill Acquisition in Nursing

P atricia Sawyer Benner was born in August, 1942, in Hampton, Virginia, to Shirley and Clint Sawyer. Her father was a shipbuilder, and she was the middle child with one sister older and one younger than she. Her family moved to Ontario, California, where the Sawyer girls completed their high school education. Her parents divorced when she was a sophomore in high school, which she reported as a very difficult time for all of them. She became interested in becoming a nurse when she worked as an admitting clerk at Saint Luke's Hospital while in college. The college she was attending, Pasadena College, did not offer nursing as a major, so she transferred to Pasadena City College, where she obtained her associate of science in nursing degree while simultaneously receiving a bachelor's degree in 1964 from Pasadena College. She went on to earn a master's degree in nursing from the University of California at San Francisco in 1970 and a PhD at the University of California at Berkeley in 1982.

Benner was one of only a few nurse theorists who married and had children. She married Richard Benner in August 1967, and according to Dr. Benner, her husband's study of situational leadership had a profound effect on her understanding of practice. She has two children, a son born in 1973, and a daughter born in 1981 (Alligood, n.d.).

Benner has worked as a professor of nursing at the University of California–San Francisco (UCSF) since 1982. Benner was the first to hold the Thelma Shobe Endowed Chair in Ethics and Spirituality position at the UCSF; she held the position from 2002 until 2008. She is a fellow of the American Academy of Nursing. Since 2004, Benner has served as the director of the Carnegie Foundation's Preparation for the Profession Program. This work focuses on nursing schools' role in the education of nurses. The findings of this research were published in a book entitled *Educating Nurses: A Call for Radical Transformation* in December of 2009.

Theoretical Influences

Benner readily acknowledges that her work in model development has been influenced by a number of individuals, including nurse theorist Virginia Henderson and University of California–Berkeley professors Hubert and Stuart Dreyfus, as well as the work of existential philosophers Richard Heidegger, Soren Kierkegaard, and Maurice Merleau-Ponty (Tomey & Alligood, 2006).

Benner studied clinical nursing in an attempt to uncover new knowledge but was very careful to emphasize that practical knowledge without theoretical understanding is problematic. While Benner worked in California, she was introduced to the skill acquisition work of philosopher Hubert Dreyfus and his younger brother, Stuart Dreyfus, an operational engineer. Benner found that skill acquisition is very applicable to nursing. The Dreyfuses' model was developed by studying the processes experts used to play chess, as well as armored tank drivers' and airplane pilots' performances in emergency situations.

The Dreyfuses' model is situational and identifies the following five levels of skill acquisition: novice, advanced beginner, competent, proficient, and expert. Movement from one level to the next occurs in several ways. One way is the movement from reliance on abstract principles to the use of past concrete experience as paradigms. The second is a change in the learner's perception of the situation, where the situation is seen less and less as a mass of equally relevant bits, and more and more as a complete whole where only certain parts are relevant. The third is a passage from detached observation to involved performer. The performer no longer stands outside the situation but is now engaged in the situation.

Model of Skill Acquisition

Benner adapted the Dreyfuses' model to clinical nursing and in 1984 published her classic book *From Novice to Expert: Excellence and Power in Clinical Nursing Practice*, where she outlined her model of skill acquisition in nursing. Based on the development of skills outlined by Dreyfus and Dreyfus (1980), Benner was able to describe the process by which nurses learn to practice nursing.

Benner (1984) distinguishes between theoretical knowledge, "knowing that," and practical knowledge, "knowing how," by stating that knowledge development in a practice discipline comes from extending how to do something through scientific investigation based on theory. Benner believes that practical knowledge can extend knowledge and that clinical practice is a rich source for knowledge development. Benner believes that a nurse can be knowledgeable and skillful without ever knowing the theory.

In Benner's model, she identifies seven domains of nursing practice. They are the helping role, teaching-coaching function, diagnostic-patient monitoring function, effective management of rapidly changing situations, administration and monitoring of therapeutic interventions and regimens, monitoring and ensuring the quality of healthcare practices, and organizational and work role competencies (Benner, 1984).

In 1989, Benner extended her model by introducing the concept of caring as a response to stress. Benner worked with Dr. Judith Wrubel on the identification of the existence of caring and its integration into the process of skill acquisition (Benner & Wrubel, 1989).

Skill Acquisition in Nursing

Stage 1: Novice

The first stage of skill acquisition is the novice. In nursing, Benner views novices as beginners, usually students in undergraduate nursing programs, who have no experience with the types of situations in which they are expected to perform. Novices are taught rules to help them perform. The rules are context free and independent of specific cases; hence the rules tend to be rigidly applied in all situations. The rule-governed behavior typical of the novice is extremely limited and inflexible. As such, novices have no life experience in the application of rules. Rules can't tell a novice which tasks to perform in which situations, so behavior in the clinical setting is limited and inflexible, and the novice is oftentimes unable to make the leap from classroom to practice.

Stage 2: Advanced Beginner

Advanced beginners have had enough experiences to discern recurring, meaningful patterns in a situation or to have had them pointed out by a mentor. This usually occurs during the first 6 months after graduation from nursing school. Advanced beginners are beginning to create their own guidelines that can determine their actions. They can perform at a minimal level in real situations. According to Benner (1984), they possess the knowledge, skills, and understanding but lack the in-depth encounters in population.

Stage 3: Competent

After approximately 2–3 years of nursing practice, the competent nurse begins to see the long-term effect of his or her actions in patient situations; however he or she lacks the efficiency and adaptability seen in proficient nurses. Competent nurses do have a feeling of mastery and can plan and organize effectively. An increasing ability to recognize the salient or most important adds to their effectiveness. They begin to recognize patterns and are able to interpret clinical situations more quickly and accurately.

Stage 4: Proficient

The proficient nurse is able to learn from experiences the expected outcome in a given situation and how one should alter plans in response to events. In the proficient stage of the Dreyfuses' model, nurses view situations in their entirety rather than the component parts. Principles and maxims guide the proficient nurse. The proficient nurse learns from past experiences what events typically occur and how to modify plans in response to different events. The proficient nurse is able to recognize when the expected outcome does not occur. The proficient nurse is able to detect the most important events and subtle nuances and is able to intervene when necessary. This holistic understanding improves the proficient nurse's decision making; however, she must still consciously make decisions. Proficiency usually manifests after 3–4 years of clinical practice.

Stage 5: Expert

The expert performer no longer relies on rules or maxims to make the connection of a situation and needed appropriate intervention. The expert nurse has an intuitive grasp of situations and is able to focus quickly on the correct problem. The expert operates from a deep understanding of the total situation. Experts use rules, guidelines, and maxims only when confronted with a new and unique event. Nurses usually become experts after 5 or more years of clinical practice; however, some nurses never reach expert clinical performance, according to Benner (1984).

Concepts

Benner and Wrubel expanded the model of skill acquisition in nursing by including the concept of caring in nursing practice. Benner and Wrubel defined and described the concepts of caring, nursing, person, health, stress, coping, and situation in a 1989 publication, *The Primacy of Caring: Stress and Coping in Health and Illness*, and used examples of nurse–patient interactions to illustrate the processes and concepts.

Caring

Caring is defined as being connected and having things matter, with fused thoughts, feelings, and action. Caring sets up what is important to a person, and therefore it sets up what is stressful and how a person might cope. Benner and Wrubel (1989) state that all caring rises from connectedness and having some things matter more than others. "Without care, a person would be without projects and concerns. Care ... sets up meaning distinctions" (Benner & Wrubel, 1989, p. 1).

The behaviors related to caring are characterized by empathy, support, compassion, protection, and nurturance. When a nurse cares for a client, that care creates stress because it is an emotional investment, an engagement process. Engaging with clients makes it possible for nurses to diagnose problems and identify solutions and create a trusting environment. Caring is of primary importance, according to Benner and Wrubel, because it creates the environment where the nurse is able to provide assistance to the client (1989).

Care is primary because it:

- sets up what matters, what is stressful, what options are possible to cope
- creates an enabling condition of connection and concern
- sets up the possibility of giving and getting help (Benner & Wrubel, 1989)

Nursing

Nursing is described as a relationship based on caring in an "enabling condition of connection and concern" (Benner & Wrubel, 1989, p. 4). Nursing science is guided by the art and ethics of care and responsibility. "Nurses promote healing through assisting the patient to maintain human ties and concerns and it is the human connection that gives people the courage to weather their illness" (Benner & Wrubel, 1989, p. 87). The relationship of health, illness, and disease is central to Benner and Wrubel's view of nursing practice.

Person

Benner and Wrubel's interpretation of *person* is based on existential philosophy and the oneness or wholeness of human beings. Benner thus describes person as "a self-interpreting being, that is, the person does not come into the world predefined but gets defined in the course of living a life" (p. 41). A person is viewed as a creative, generative being who lives in the context of meaning and whose actions and understandings form a comprehensible whole. Benner and

Wrubel characterize the person as someone who must deal with situations, body, personal concerns, and the temporary nature of events (1989).

Health

Benner and Wrubel use Kleinman, Eisenberg, and Good's definition of health as "health [is] not the absence of illness and illness is not identical with disease" (1989, p. 8). Illness is described as the experience of loss or dysfunction, whereas disease is the manifestation of aberration at the cellular, tissue, or organ level. All treatment for disease and illness must make sense within the context of the lived human experience.

Situation

Benner uses situation, rather than the concept of environment, in her work. Benner chose situation because, according to Benner, situation has a social context with meaning and interpretation, which impacts people. People "inhabit their world, rather than live in an environment" (Benner & Wrubel, 1989, p. 49). A person's interpretation impacts each situation. Benner's phenomenologically based view of situation is evident in her writing when she uses the terms *being situated* and *situated meaning*, indicating a person's engagement with and interpretation of each life event.

Stress

According to Benner and Wrubel, stress is "the disruption of meanings, understanding, and smooth functioning so that harm, loss, or challenge is experienced, and sorrow, interpretation, or new skill acquisition is required" (1989, p. 59). Stress is viewed as the physical, emotional, and/or intellectual realization that smooth functioning has been disrupted. Stress occurs when the person understands that something is amiss or out of balance. Stress is the inevitable consequence of living in a world where one cares about things, and therefore it cannot be eliminated.

Coping

Coping is not considered an antidote for stress but rather what one does about the disruption caused by the stress. Benner and Wrubel draw on the work of Lazarus (1966) to explain stress and coping. Coping is "doing something directly" as well as "not doing something on purpose" (Benner & Wrubel, 1989, p. 62). Other coping behaviors are seeking information, reframing the way one views the situation, and making a choice to have a positive attitude in the face of the disruption. Benner and Wrubel give numerous examples of how one copes with various situations such as development across the life span, caregiving itself, various symptoms, cancer, and neurologic illnesses, among others (1989).

Summary

Benner's work on skill acquisition and stress, coping, and caring offers insight into these complex and important issues derived directly from nursing practice. While some have criticized Benner's work of the "intuitive knower" as leading to subjective understanding of nursing knowledge without empirical validation and her form of phenomenologic understanding of nursing practice, the Benner model can help nurses understand how expertise develops, allowing them to support and nurture each other (Reed & Shearer, 2009). Benner's work on skill acquisition has been extremely helpful to nurse educators and administrators in knowing more about how students and nurses learn and advance in their knowledge over their careers, and her work with Wrubel on caring represents a totally new view of this central concept.

Benner's model has led to the development of nursing competencies in multiple domains and expanded to reflect advanced practice and critical care nursing (Benner, 1984; Benner, Hooper-Kyriakidis, & Stannard, 1999; Brykczynski, 1999). Benner's work also validated the value of narrative accounts of nursing in expanding nursing knowledge and the central role of caring in the practice of nursing.

Learning Activities

1. Think of the first time you were to give a hospitalized patient a bed bath. Recall the preparation for that task. Now compare it to giving a patient a bed bath today. Discuss the growth you have experienced in your skill level.
2. Recall nurses you have seen caring for different patients. Give examples of situations where a nurse noticed a subtle change in a patient's condition that you had overlooked and reflect on what clues the nurse must have noticed that you did not pick up on.
3. One of Benner's assumptions is that all caring rises from connectedness and having some things matter more than others. Do you agree or disagree, and why?

Web Sites

http://nurseweb.ucsf.edu/www/ffbennp.htm

>   Patricia Benner's faculty profile.

http://www.bennerassociates.com/ci_patriciabenner.html

>   Benner's consulting firm.

http://socrates.berkeley.edu/~hdreyfus/

>   Homepage for Dr. Hubert Dreyfus, emeriti professor, 2009–2010, University of California–Berkley.

Theories that Defy Classification

PART

V

Envisioning Theories That Defy Classification Through Space Photography

"Theories That Defy Classification" is not a phrase traditionally used to describe nursing theories. Martha Rogers's Unitary Human Beings and Margaret Newman's Health as Expanding Consciousness are discussed in this section of the text because they are both unusually progressive and ground breaking. The concepts proposed in these theories broadly encompass facets of philosophy, theoretical physics, spirituality, health/wellness, wholism, nondualism, and alternative approaches to understanding the universe. Because of the ongoing theoretical exploration and boundary testing associated with these theories, it is not possible to place them in any of the three traditional classifications previously discussed. These same attributes have made them somewhat difficult to understand, controversial, and not directly applicable to practice.

However, these theories are valuable to the nursing profession because they challenge traditional thinking, spawn professional debate, and provide fresh possibilities for future conceptualizations of nursing.

Envision space photography when exploring nursing theories that defy classification. When trying to understand such theories, one can envision space photography, noting its nebulous, undefined nature. Photos of the cosmos taken with telescopes convey boundlessness and the notion of a new frontier, much like Rogers's and Newman's theories. The Hubble Space Telescope has taken thousands of stunning photographs of space, reaching into the far corners of the universe (see Color Plates 21.1 and 21.2 in the color insert).

No matter from how far away the images come, there is still more beyond to reach out to—the unending darkness and glowing shapes just out of focusing range of the camera. Theories that defy classification are much the same; they propose new, limitless perceptions of nursing and humanity, and have philosophical boundaries that are blurry and ever expanding.

Perform a Web search using the phrase *Hubble Space Telescope*. Visit one of a number of sites with Hubble Space Telescope galleries that offer photographs for viewing. Envision these photographs as visual representations of progressive theories that challenge the traditional boundaries of accepted thinking and reasoning in nursing and health care.

When exploring theories that defy classification, ask these questions:

1. What aspects of humanity are explored in the theory?
2. What are the central concepts that form the basis of the theory?
3. Is there an overall theme that governs perceptions of the central concepts?
4. How might the propositions expressed in this theory affect everyday nursing practice?
5. Does the theory resonate with your own experience?

Learning Activities

1. Perform an Internet search using the phrase *Hubble Space Telescope* to find stunning photographs of outer space taken from the Hubble Space Telescope. Print four of your favorite photos and paste them onto the blank pages at the end of the chapter.
2. Go to the Jones and Bartlett Web site for this text at *http://nursing.jbpub.com* and explore the Web links listed for this chapter.

Feel free to use these blank pages as a canvas for your learning activities.

Martha Rogers's Unitary Human Beings

M artha Rogers (1914–1994) was born in Dallas, Texas. She received her diploma in nursing from Knoxville, Tennessee, General Hospital School of Nursing in 1936. She earned her B.S. in nursing from George Peabody College in Nashville, Tennessee, in 1937. Rogers earned an M.A. in public health nursing supervision in 1954 from Teachers College, Columbia University, New York. She then earned a master's degree in public health (M.P.H.) in 1952 and an Sc.D. in 1954 from Johns Hopkins University in Baltimore. Rogers's early nursing practice was in the area of rural community health nursing. From 1954 to 1975, she was professor and head of the division of nursing at New York University. After 1975, Rogers was a professor at New York University, becoming Professor Emerita in 1979. She held this title until her death at the age of 79 (Tomey & Alligood, 2002). Over her long career, Rogers published more than 200 articles and 3 books. She also received many awards for her contributions to nursing.

Rogers was a nurse visionary who created an innovative conceptual system that continues to impact the nursing profession today. Rogers's model is supported by continued development of similar ideas associated with chaos theory and quantum physics. Rogers loved the color purple and dreamed of nursing in space. She created an innovative conceptual system that views humans as energy fields identified by patterns.

The first question in discussing Rogers's Unitary Human Beings might be: What does the word unitary mean? Rogers used the word *unitary* to describe human beings as intrinsically whole rather than a sum of parts. Information about physiological functioning or a person's social background may be helpful in providing care; however, this information does not impart full understanding of the unitary human being. In order to understand Rogers's concepts, it becomes necessary to shift one's perception from viewing a client as the sum of many parts to viewing the client and his/her environment as infinite energy fields with no physical boundaries.

Nine assertions about the nature of humankind and human life form the basis of Unitary Human Beings (Biley, 2002; Toomey & Alligood, 2002):

1. *Wholeness* refers to when a person is thought of as being different and more than a sum of parts.
2. *Openness* describes the continual interchange of matter and energy between the individual and the environment.
3. *Unidirectionality* describes the assertion that the life process is not reversible, similar to a car driving down a one-way street that cannot back up.
4. *Pattern and organization* identifies individuals and reflects fluid, ever-changing wholeness.
5. *Sentience and thought* is a human trait—human beings being the only living creatures capable of imagination, abstraction, language, thought, sensation, and emotion.
6. *One energy field* that is infinite constitutes all matter, both living and nonliving. There are two kinds of fields: the human field and the environmental field.
7. *Universe of open systems* describes infinite groups of energy fields that interact with one another continuously.
8. *Patterns* define unique energy fields. Patterns change continuously, giving identity to human environmental energy fields.
9. *The pandimension* is an infinite domain and contains all energy fields. It fully represents the unitary whole.

Basic definitions of three key terms may be helpful in clarifying specific concepts (Biley, 2002):

- A *person* is more than a sum of parts, and it is impossible to divide a person into parts and still be able to understand the whole person.

- The *environment* is a wave pattern. The pattern changes continuously. Each human field pattern is unique and is seamlessly intertwined with its own unique environmental field pattern.
- *Nursing* is an organized body of abstract knowledge, used for the purpose of "assisting human beings to move in the direction of maximum well-being" (Rogers, 1994, p. 64).

Rogers did not specifically mention the notions of *health, wellness,* or *illness* in her writings. Many scholars believe that this is because levels of illness and wellness are based on social definitions and probably encourage the tendency to view a person as a "sum of parts" rather than as a unitary being.

Nursing actions based on Rogers's Unitary Human Beings include (Cowling, 1990):

1. Interventions that arise from the nurse's awareness of continuously interacting energy fields based on patterns rather than age, disease process, gender, or other factors
2. Awareness of the influence of individual perceptions, experiences, and modes of expression
3. Actions based on all modes of sentient awareness including the five senses and also intuition, feelings, thoughts, imagination, memories, and any other expressions of human awareness
4. Pattern recognition involving all human ways of knowing that is continuous and based in reality
5. Assessments communicated verbally or through visual input
6. Assessments created by the nurse that are either accepted or not accepted by the client
7. Interventions based on mutual nurse and client acceptance of assessments
8. Ongoing evaluation and reevaluation of assessments and actions with continual input from self, environment, and client

In summary, Rogers's innovative approach to understanding humanity, and nursing's place in it, has illuminated new horizons of inquiry within all nursing practice settings (George, 2002). Within the framework of Rogers's Unitary Human Beings, the function of nursing becomes that of recognizing patterns of energy within client and self and then mutually acting to guide and redirect these patterns to support optimum functioning. Rogers broadened the concept of wholism in nursing by essentially removing the notion that a "whole" entity must be composed of a grouping of parts and asserting that all things are intrinsically whole and seamlessly connected with all that is. In 1966, Rogers wrote the following about nursing:

> Nursing's story is a magnificent epic of service to mankind. It is about people: How they are born, and live, and die; in health and in sickness; in joy and in sorrow. Its mission is the translation of knowledge into human service.

> Nursing is compassionate concern for human beings. It is the heart that understands and the hand that soothes. It is the intellect that synthesizes many learnings into meaningful ministrations (Rogers, 1966, cited in Barrett, 1990, p. 31).

Here is one way to visualize a Rogerian universe: Envision outer space, a black limitless background without boundary. Orbs of light appear at various depths. Some of the orbs are bright white, others a cool blue or green, and still others are yellow, red, and orange. Superimpose over this entire universe a finely woven, four-dimensional matrix made of extremely fine silver thread. Each of the orbs in this universe exists in, around, and through the netting. Envision the net and all it contains flexing, undulating, and alternately becoming dense and thin in an unending dance of interaction and movement. None of what makes up this universe disappears, and no new entities appear. There is just gentle shifting of movement and the gradual, irreversible transformation of orbs and netting in a continual journey of manifest completeness.

Learning Activities

1. Answer the following questions about Rogers's theory:
   a. What aspects of humanity are explored in the theory?
   b. What are the central concepts that form the basis of the theory?
   c. Is there an overall theme that governs perceptions of the central concepts?
   d. How might the propositions expressed in this theory affect everyday nursing practice?
   e. Does the theory resonate with your own experience?

2. Perform an Internet search using the phrase *Hubble Space Telescope* to find stunning photographs of outer space taken from the Hubble Space Telescope. Print your favorite photo to represent Rogers's theory and paste it onto page 184 to share with classmates.

3. Find Web sites or journal articles about Rogers's theory. Words to use when performing a search might include:
   - Martha Rogers
   - Unitary Human Beings
   - Rogerian

4. Go to the Jones and Bartlett Web site for this text at *http://nursing.jbpub.com* and explore the Web links listed for this chapter.

Feel free to use these blank pages as a canvas for your learning activities.

Margaret Newman's Health as Expanding Consciousness

M argaret Newman was born in Memphis, Tennessee, in 1933. She earned a B.S.H.E. in Home Economics and English from Baylor University in Texas in 1954. After caring for her mother during a terminal illness, Newman decided to become a nurse. She earned a B.S. in nursing from the University of Memphis in 1962 and an M.S. in nursing from the University of California in San Francisco in 1964. In 1971, she earned a Ph.D. in nursing science and rehabilitation from New York University. Newman taught at the University of Tennessee, New York University, and Pennsylvania State University. She retired from the University of Minnesota in 1996. She has received many awards for nursing leadership and scholarship.

Newman's Health as Expanding Consciousness was influenced by Martha Rogers (Tomey & Alligood, 2002). Newman (2003) writes:

> The theory of health as expanding consciousness stems from Rogers' theory of Unitary Human Beings. Rogers' assumptions regarding patterning of persons in interaction with the environment are basic to the view that consciousness is a manifestation of an evolving pattern of person–environment interaction . . . . Consciousness includes not only the cognitive and affective awareness normally associated with consciousness, but also the interconnectedness of the entire living system, which includes physiochemical maintenance and growth processes as well

as the immune system. This pattern of information, which is the consciousness of the system, is part of a larger, undivided pattern of an expanding universe.

Implicit in Newman's theory is the assumption that human beings have the following characteristics. According to Newman, they are (Marchione, 1993; George, 2002):

- Open energy systems
- In continual interconnectedness with a universe of open systems (environment)
- Continuously active in evolving their own pattern of the whole (health)
- Intuitive as well as affective cognitive beings
- Capable of abstract thinking as well as sensation
- More than the sum of their parts

According to Newman (2003), when the concept of health is viewed as a wholistic pattern, illness is an expression emanating from the interaction between the client and the environment. When nurses view illness in this way, then the usual focus on treatment of symptoms shifts to a focus on pattern recognition. Illness is viewed as part of the organizing process of expanding consciousness. One of the primary roles of the nurse becomes to help patients recognize and positively address their own patterns.

The focus of Newman's approach for nurses is to (George, 2002):

- Attend to the "we" in a human-to-human exchange, rather than viewing the other person as an object outside of ourselves.
- Attend to the meaning of the whole rather than the "fixing" of a part or the sum of the parts.
- Process the experience of interaction in partnership with the client.
- Cultivate compassionate mutual consciousness rather than manipulation, or control, of another person's behavior.
- Mindfully attend to the here and now (the moment) rather than try to identify past causes or possible future effects.

Newman skillfully weaves the elusive threads of this approach together with her words. About individuals, families, and communities, Newman says this:

A human being can be viewed as a center of consciousness that is continually expanding. Through knowledge of this consciousness, it is possible to sense that each life is part of a much larger whole. A single person is a pattern of consciousness, surrounded by a family pattern, then a community pattern, a world pattern, and then other endless patterns, all making an infinite whole (Newman, 2000).

Health is a process of expanding consciousness. Humans are uniquely capable of gaining insight into their own patterns of life and health. All experiences related to health, illness, and death are part of the experience of progressing to a higher level of consciousness (Newman, 2000).

Nurses intervene and provide care by forming a partnership with the client. Partnerships include trust and immediacy and result in each participant reaching a higher level of consciousness (Newman, 2000).

Here is one way to visualize Newman's Health as Expanding Consciousness: Envision a nurse and a client in a room standing a few feet away from one another. Each person is surrounded and permeated by light. Unique layers of different colored lights are moving around, within, and through each person. As the nurse and client shift toward and then away from one another in the course of an authentic caring exchange, the layers of color surrounding each person become mixed, creating new colors at every interchange. Ripples of soft light emanate from the doorway as people pass by or linger to convey greetings. The success of the exchange between nurse and client is apparent when the layers of light surrounding each gently expand outward to mingle yet further with each other and the surrounding light.

Learning Activities

1. Answer the following questions about Newman's theory:
   a. What aspects of humanity are explored in the theory?
   b. What are the central concepts that form the basis of the theory?
   c. Is there an overall theme that governs perceptions of the central concepts?
   d. How might the propositions expressed in this theory affect everyday nursing practice?
   e. Does the theory resonate with your own experience?
2. Perform an Internet search using the phrase *Hubble Space Telescope* to find stunning photographs of outer space taken from the Hubble

Space Telescope. Print your favorite photo to represent Newman's theory and paste it onto page 191 to share with classmates.

3. Find Web sites or journal articles about Newman's theory. Words to use when performing a search might include:
   - Margaret Newman
   - Health as Expanding Consciousness

4. Go to the Jones and Bartlett Web site for this text at *http://nursing.jbpub.com* and explore the Web links listed for this chapter.

Feel free to use these blank pages as a canvas for your learning activities.

Rosemarie Rizzo Parse—Theory of Human Becoming

Rosemarie Rizzo Parse was born in Pittsburgh, Pennsylvania (Reed & Shearer, 2009). Dr. Parse grew up in Castle Shannon, Pennsylvania, in a warm and supportive family. Her father was the oldest of seven children and worked with his father as a lamplighter and later became a borough manager for Castle Shannon. Her mother was a homemaker and a very active member of the local Catholic church. Parse has two siblings, an older sister, Nancy, who is also a nurse, and a brother named Frank. Her family emphasized education and the arts, and Parse took piano and dancing lessons while growing up. Parse was raised a strict Catholic and describes her childhood as wonderful. Parse states that she enjoyed school and was a very good student.

After graduating from a Catholic high school, she attended Duquesne University in Pittsburgh, where she earned her bachelor's degree in nursing. Against the advice of the dean and faculty at Duquesne, she accepted a fellowship and immediately went on to work on her master's degree in nursing at the University of Pittsburgh. When she graduated in 2 years from Pitt, according to her husband, John Parse, she became the youngest person in the United States to hold a master's degree in nursing. She went on to earn a PhD from the University of Pittsburgh while teaching at her alma mater, Duquesne. At Duquesne, she became the first woman elected to chair the faculty senate and the first dean of nursing to hold a PhD (Alligood, Krivicich, Kramer, Erickson, & Mishel, 2008).

Parse served as dean of nursing at Duquesne from 1983 to 1993 and professor and Niehoff chair at Loyola University from 1993 to 2006. Since 2007, she has served as a consultant and visiting scholar at New York University. Parse founded the Institute of Human Becoming and the journal, *Nursing Science Quarterly*, and she still serves as the journal's editor. At the *Nursing Science Quarterly*, Parse oversees a very important venue for the discussion and debate of nursing research and theory. More information about Parse can be found at *http://www.humanbecoming.org/site/default.html and http://www.discovery internationalonline.com*.

The Theory of Human Becoming

Parse describes the beginning of her theory of human becoming originating from her childhood and the values instilled in her by her parents and growing over time. The dignity of every human being was very important to her, and she described the conflict she experienced when trying to understand and use the biophysical-medical model as a framework for practice. So she began searching for a model that matched her own worldview, which led to the creation of her own nursing theory.

Parse's theory of human becoming was known as the man/living/health model when it was first published in 1981. In 1992, the theory's name was changed to human becoming to better reflect its focus on mankind without gender distinction. Parse's theory is similar to that of Martha Rogers's theory of unitary human being, and both are often referred to as simultaneity theories because they focus on a unitary human where the whole is different than the sum of its parts and cannot be understood by knowledge of the parts.

Parse read widely in the field of psychology and philosophy in addition to nursing and readily acknowledges the philosophical sources of her theory as being Martha Rogers's science of unitary human being and existential philosophers, Soren Kierkegaard, Franz Kafka, Martin Heidegger, Jean-Paul Sartre, and Maurice Merleau-Ponty (Reed, Shearer, & Nicoll, 2004). Also, during the

1960s and 70s when Parse studied at Duquesne University, the university was regarded by some as the center of the existential-phenomenological movement, and Parse was heavily influenced by this school of thought while she studied there (Parse, 1981).

Basic Beliefs/Assumptions

Many of Parse's major assumptions come from Rogers's science of unitary human beings (1970, 1992) and the existential philosophers. Parse believes that human beings are intentional; they choose and assign meaning to events, and like Rogers, she believes that human beings cannot be reduced to component parts and be fully understood. Parse's main belief is that human beings coauthor their becoming along with the universe cocreating distinct patterns. Parse also believes that human beings have free choice and cocreate health together with the universe. Therefore the human must be viewed as an expert on his or her own health and lived experiences (Parse, 1995). Parse's use of "co" means together with and is used extensively in her work.

Parse's theory includes nine assumptions, which are as follows:

1. The human is coexisting while coconstituting rhythmical patterns in the universe.
2. The human is an open being, freely choosing meaning in situation, bearing responsibility for decisions.
3. The human is a living unity continuously coconstituting patterns of relating.
4. The human is transcending multidimensionally with the possibilities.
5. Becoming is an open process experienced by the human.
6. Becoming is a rhythmically coconstituting human–universe process.
7. Becoming is the human's pattern of relating value priorities.
8. Becoming is an intersubjective process of transcending with the possibilities.
9. Becoming is human evolving (Parse, 1998, pp. 5–6).

Parse's theory includes three assumptions about human becoming, which are:

1. Human becoming is freely choosing personal meaning in a situation in the intersubjective process of relating value priorities.

2. Human becoming is cocreating rhythmic patterns of relating in open process with the universe.
3. Human becoming is cotranscending multidimensionally with the emerging possible (Parse, 1992, p. 38).

The four main components of Parse's theory are the mutual process of the human universe, the coconstitution of health, the multidimensional meanings the indivisible human gives to being and becoming, and the human's freedom in situations to choose alternative paths of becoming.

Parse asserts that the human is coexisting while coconstituting rhythmic patterns with the environment. Coexistence means that humans are not alone in any "dimension of becoming" (Parse, 1998, p. 17). To create her nine assumptions, Parse pulled from Rogers's principles of helicy, integrality, and resonancy; her concepts of energy field, openness, pattern, and four dimensionality; as well as major constructs found in existential philosophy (Reed, Shearer, & Nicoll, 2004). The theory of human becoming is the only nursing theory that regards paradoxes as an integral part of the human experience. Paradoxes are normal in life and, according to Parse, should not be viewed as a problem to be solved.

Parse's theory is based on three main themes or concepts entitled meaning, rhythmicity, and transcendence. Each of these themes gives rise to additional concepts where structuring meaning relates to the concepts of imagining, valuing, and languaging; the concept of rhythmicity relates to revealing-concealing, enabling-limiting, and connecting-separating; and the concept of transcendence relates to powering, originating, and transforming.

Principles

Parse outlines three principles in her theory that she indicates flow from her theoretical assumptions. Each of the three principles has three component concepts subsumed under the principles. The three principles are:

Principle 1—Structuring meaning multidimensionally is cocreating reality through the languaging of valuing and imaging (Parse, 1998, p. 35). Component concepts are imaging, valuing, and languaging.

Principle 2—Cocreating rhythmic patterns of relating is living the paradoxic unity of revealing-concealing and enabling-limiting while connecting-separating (Parse, 1998, p. 42). Component concepts are revealing-concealing, enabling-limiting, and connecting-separating.

Principle 3—Cotranscending with the possible is powering unique ways of originating in the process of transforming (Parse, 1998, p. 46). Component concepts are powering, originating, and transforming. Structuring meaning explains that humans choose the meaning of their own realities, and the choosing that occurs is not always a conscious undertaking. This explains why people lack insight into their behavior oftentimes. Imaging, valuing, and languaging are component concepts within the principle of structuring. Imaging is how a person sees his or her own reality, valuing is the process by which a person confirms his or her beliefs, and languaging is the process by which humans express their reality. Languaging can occur with words or symbols or by using nonverbal signals, movement, etc. (Parse, 1981, 1998).

Cocreating is the second principle and involves the process that humans use to express their personal values and meanings through the creation of patterns. Cocreation means that people live in rhythm with the universe. It is about choices, connections, and letting go. The concepts embedded in cocreating are revealing-concealing, enabling-limiting, and connecting-separating. Revealing-concealing is the process humans use to show or hide their personal evolution or becoming. It involves how much we want to share about ourselves with others. Enabling-limiting refers to the opportunities or restrictions that occur daily. Humans are confronted with opportunities every moment, and choices are made whether to act upon the chance or not. Enabling-limiting is about making choices and living with the consequences of actions. Connecting-separating is a description of the creation of patterns through the processes of connecting and separating with people, things, and places. Connecting and separating is about joining with and separating from something (Parse, 1981, 1998).

Cotranscending is about humans engaging with and choosing how to be and the attitudes and approaches one selects. Powering, originating, and transforming are the concepts that make up the principle of cotranscending. Powering is the concept that relates the struggle humans display when confronted with hardships and threats. Powering is a push-pull process that is always occurring. Originating is about the uniqueness of humans. Humans seek to be original and stand apart from others and yet at the same time feel the need to blend in. This sense of being unique and needing to be like others causes certainty and uncertainty. Transforming is the third concept in cotranscending and is about creating deliberate change and the way humans view themselves. Transforming is a continuous process of evolution as humans seek to understand the changes occurring (Parse, 1981, 1998).

Nursing

Parse does not write about nursing as a concept in her theory; however, she refers to the core of nursing science and nursing's focus of concern as the human-universe-health process, which, according to Parse, is the basic interrelationship of the human, the universe, and health (Parse, 1992). Parse believes that quality of life is the goal of nursing. The belief that human beings are free to choose is fundamental to the practice of nursing with all actions focused on guiding humans toward ways of being, finding meaning, and choosing ways of cocreating their own health (Parse, 1995, 1998). Parse also writes about requirements that she believes are essential for nursing practice, which are:

- possessing the knowledge and use of nursing frameworks and theories
- offering of self
- valuing others
- respecting differences
- taking accountability for one's actions
- desiring to experience and test that which is new and unknown
- connecting with others
- being proud of oneself
- liking what one does
- recognizing the joy and struggles in living
- appreciating mystery and newness
- being competent
- having a willingness to rest and begin again (Parse, 1989)

Human-Universe-Health Process

According to Parse, human, universe, and health are concepts that cannot be viewed separately, and while they can be described individually, they are always linked together (Parse, 1990, 1996, 1998). Parse refers to health as a "cocreated process of becoming as experienced and described by the person, family and community" (Parse, 1989, p. 11). Health is a way of being in the world—not a continuum with health and illness at opposite ends but rather a day-to-day way of being. Health is a personal commitment with ebbs and flows.

Human beings can be described as intentional, knowing beings who are involved with their world, open to their world and cocreating meaning in multidimensional mutual process with the universe. This mutual process with the universe can be recognized by patterns of relating and the ability to freely choose. Parse believes that human beings have responsibility for their health. Parse views the universe as the world and those who occupy spaces along with others who freely choose to be in the situation (Parse, 1998). Like Rogers, Parse sees the human and the environment or universe as mutually and simultaneously interrelated and believes that the human-universe-health process is more than the sum of its parts and health as ever changing (Parse, 1987).

Summary

Parse's theory of human becoming is considered a grand theory that focuses on the irreducibility of human beings and the interrelationship between human beings and the universe. While complex and somewhat difficult to understand because of the terminology and the abstractness of her concepts, Parse's writing offers a framework from which to view the patterns of human lived experiences. The perspective brought to nursing by the human becoming theory is a very important one with human beings being viewed as intentional, with the right to freely choose and more than the sum of the component parts. No doubt as more and more nurses use the theory in practice and in research, the theory of human becoming will continue to offer a perspective of possibilities.

Learning Activities

1. Choose one of Parse's concepts, such as meaning, valuing, languaging, or revealing-concealing and explain how it might be used to interpret a client's behavior.
2. Explain how denial often seen in clients with alcoholism might be interpreted using Parse's concepts.
3. Suggest some nursing interventions that would be consistent with Parse's theory and in what type of care scenario they might be used.
4. Discuss one idea or concept expressed by Parse that caused you to think more deeply about a client situation you might have encountered. How would your approach to your client have been different if viewed through Parse's theory of human becoming?

Web Sites

http://library.loyno.edu/services_collections/streaming/?id=34

   Streaming video of interview with Dr. Parse

http://www.humanbecoming.org

http://nsq.sagepub.com/

http://www.discoveryinternationalonline.com

Feel free to use these blank pages as a canvas for your learning activities.

Conclusion

PART
VI

CHAPTER

27

Further Development of Nursing Theory

Theories about nursing are as varied as nurses themselves. Some nurse leaders feel that development of theory supporting evidence-based practice is where future focus should be (Evers, 2001). Many questions remain that must be formally explored and answered regarding effective nursing practice (Evers, 2001). Other nurses feel that "Nursing theories are needed that have social justice as their goal" (Drevdahl, 1999, p. 1). These nurses believe that, in the future, broad social issues will supercede other nursing concerns and create the need for theories that address environmental problems, global poverty, diminishing health status, and ethnic and religious conflicts (Drevdahl, 1999). Still others value the development of theories that explore what it means to inhabit a human body and experience issues associated with health and wellness (sentience) (Wilde, 1999). Theories are also being developed that are based on the notion that *caring* is the central concept that makes nursing a unique profession (Watson, 2003).

There are many different kinds of theories because nurses provide care to human beings and human beings are multifaceted, having physical, mental, spiritual, psychological, social, and existential elements. One theory, or one type of theory, could not begin to fully describe all that is nursing. Also, every nurse that seeks to describe nursing practice through the creation of a theory has a slightly different vantage point than any other nurse. There will always be a wide array of theories that describe the practice of nursing.

Unfortunately, there is a general sense that, within the nursing ranks, two distinct theoretical camps exist. One camp values scientific, structured inquiry over all other methods of exploring and clarifying what nursing *is* and what nurses *do*. The other camp values narrative, personalized inquiry (Glazer, 2000). This division is not necessary because both kinds of theory arise from different aspects of nursing practice, and both aspects are needed in nursing. Effective nursing practice requires highly structured technical knowledge and action based on scientific inquiry and theory generation. Effective nursing practice *also* requires less structured, but equally valid, knowledge and action regarding mental, spiritual, psychological, social, and existential human experience based on narrative, personalized inquiry, and theory building. The combination of both kinds of theory forms a complete picture of the profession, and neither approach could begin to fully express all that nursing *is*.

Nursing actions are practical in nature; thus theory should guide and clarify actual practice. This creates a need for scholarly theory that has the potential to improve practice. As Cash (2001) states, "Because nursing is a practical activity, theory has to be a guide to practice, not an end in itself. In other words, the concepts to be clarified have to be relevant to clinical practice in some way and conclusions reached lead to some new or changed action (p. 2)." All of the theories explored in this text have the power to change nursing practice on some level, depending on how and in what situation the theory is used.

In clarifying the need for a variety of nursing theories, a common childhood story comes to mind: One day, the king of a small kingdom went hunting with the fire chief. While they were gone, the king's palace caught fire due to an unfortunate kitchen mishap. Because the fire chief was out hunting with the king, the volunteer fire department did not mobilize to put the fire out, and the whole palace burned to the ground. Upon the king's return, it was mandated that every adult in the kingdom should abandon their chosen profession and become a firefighter so that the palace would never burn down again. After a week of no bakery goods, no fresh produce, no clean laundry or dishes, no babysitters, no school teachers, no construction workers, and no police, the king realized that it takes more than firefighters to effectively run a kingdom. He mandated that everyone return to their old jobs. The moral of the story: It takes all kinds to effectively run a kingdom (or in this case, the nursing profession).

The key to progress with respect to theory generation lies in the ability of nurses and nursing leaders to appreciate the unique value in a variety of approaches, even when some approaches do not resonate with every nurse. In this way, the knowledge base in the profession will continue to grow, reflecting the richness and diversity found in the nursing ranks and nursing practice.

As the profession of nursing continues to evolve, nursing theories will also evolve. More middle-range theories will be created to clarify effective nursing approaches in specific clinical areas, and there will be further clarification of how to apply nursing grand theories and philosophies. Older theories will be expanded, revisited, and explored for relevancy to today's nursing practice, and new theories will be created. Newer theories will evolve based on current practice concerns and questions that are influenced by the current healthcare and general social climate. One of the most valuable aspects of theory development in nursing is the ongoing thought, dialogue, and variety precipitated by the process. Another valuable aspect is that the continued development of theory will lead to better-informed practice for all nurses.

Learning Activity

Go to the Jones and Bartlett Web site for this text at *http://nursing.jbpub.com* and explore the Web links listed for this chapter.

Use of Information Technology by Nurse Theorists

More than 150 years ago, Nightingale wrote her thoughts with pen and ink by candlelight. Her thoughts were compiled into a small book called *Notes on Nursing*, and she began the profession of nursing (Nightingale, 1859). She planted the seeds of nursing theory with instructions for gathering nursing knowledge. It took almost 100 years for nursing to embrace the need for nursing theory and to begin again.

In 1900, the *American Journal of Nursing* was the first formal method of communicating nursing knowledge to nurses who were lucky enough to have access to it (Kalisch & Kalisch, 1995). Full-text journal articles are now available online any time on virtually any computer, as needed. Today, the creation, development, refinement, and dissemination of knowledge are radically different than just 20 years ago, and certainly different than 120 years ago. This radical change has occurred in large part because of computer and Internet technology.

With global travel, telecommunications, information technology, and the Internet, the boundaries of space, time, geography, and language have greatly diminished the barriers that nurse theorists faced in the twentieth century. Today, because of current technology, it is possible for almost any student to ask a major theorist a question about a theory and receive an answer without ever leaving his or her living room. Nurses who have an interest in nursing theory now have the opportunity to connect with colleagues internationally with similar interests that they would otherwise have never met and learn from participation in online communities.

Current Uses of Technology

Nursing theory entered cyberspace in the late 1980s and early 1990s when nurses began using e-mail and listservs, or "cyber circles," to communicate. The use of information technology resulted in a paradigm shift in the dissemination of information and in relationships among theorists.

One of the most unique characteristics of the Internet is its ability to connect millions of people instantaneously at any time. Certainly books, journals, and audio/visual media have the ability to transmit knowledge, but they do not have the ability to facilitate "community" like the Internet does. This "connectedness" has the potential to create a community that is not limited by space, time, geography, or sociopolitical issues. Connectedness is limited only by one's ability to access the Internet. The ability to connect has allowed nurses to find others with whom they share common theory and research interests. Through online discussions, chats, and listservs, nurses who have ideas and questions about theories have the opportunity to seek feedback, support, and funding ideas. Not only do online discussions provide access to new colleagues, but computer-mediated chats allow individuals who are timid and hesitant to speak up in groups to ask questions they would never speak in public (Deering & Eichelberger, 2002).

Listservs were one of the original communication tools used by groups of nurse theorists. One of the oldest listservs is Parse-L, which was created on February 4, 1993, by Pat Lyon. It is an international discussion forum and information exchange network for Parse's Theory of Human Becoming. Dr. Parse monitors the list and occasionally responds to questions. Students often sign on to ask questions for theory assignments. The Parse-L listserv has 167 members from 17 countries (P. Lyon, personal communication sent to Lisa Eichelberger, June 6, 2003). In general, theory listservs are quite manageable and do not have as much traffic as other nursing listservs. Addresses for theory listservs can be found on the Web page for this textbook at *http://nursing.jbpub.com*.

Nursing Theory Web Sites

There are two types of theory Web sites: link sites and content sites. Link sites are composite sites where visitors can go to find links to pages on various nursing theories. In addition, these sites offer various other theory-related links, such as theory conferences, textbooks, e-mail addresses for theorists, and links to other theory-related sites.

In contrast, content sites are devoted to an individual theorist or theory. Most theorists have their own Web sites; however, some do not have any information on the Web. If you have an interest in developing Web material for a theorist who does not have a Web site, please contact *lisaeichelberger@mail. clayton.edu*. Individual Web addresses for various nurse theorists can be found on the Web page for this textbook at the Jones and Bartlett Web site.

Link Sites

The Nursing Theory Page is the original nursing theory site on the Internet and remains the premiere site for theory-related information. It is a collaborative effort by an international group of dedicated individuals who are committed to sharing nursing theory within the profession. The group seeks to develop a complete collection of resources about nursing theories throughout the world. The project began on May 21, 1996, and has played a very important part in the advancement of nursing theory. Dr. Judy Norris of the University of Alberta was the founding Webmaster and served in that capacity until May 2003 when she retired. At that time, the Webmaster duties was transferred to the Hahn School of Nursing and Health Sciences at the University of San Diego.

The Clayton College and State University (CCSU) Department of Nursing Web site began in November 1996. Tommy Thomas and Carolyn Stewart designed the basic Web site as a part of the requirements for an undergraduate nursing theory class, under the direction of Dr. Lisa Wright Eichelberger. The Theory Web Page was created to help students locate information about nursing theorists on the World Wide Web. Since 1997, Dr. Eichelberger has been the Webmaster for the site and often responds to e-mails from students from all over the world asking for information about different theorists. Unfortunately, there are still theorists for whom no information exists on the Web. (See the

CCSU Internet site for a list of theorists without a Web site). The CCSU Theory Site receives more than 1000 hits per week.

Content Sites

Most nurse theorists have some sort of Web presence, whether it be a professionally developed Web site or a link to a simple biography or obituary. (As with all content on the Web site, addresses change and links become broken, so it is important to notify a Webmaster of inactive links.) Several theorists have e-mail addresses and can be reached with a simple e-mail. Even if the theorist is deceased, individuals who are experts or historians with expert knowledge of the nurse theorist often are available and willing to assist others in learning about a particular nurse theorist. Florence Nightingale, for example, has one of the most extensive Web presences of any theorist, and a bulletin board devoted to her and her work receives about 300 hits per day during the school year, many from school-age children (J. McDonald, personal communication sent to Lisa Eichelberger, June 8, 2003).

One of the most exciting opportunities that the Internet provides is communication directly with a particular theorist. Some theory sites have chats or bulletin boards where anyone can post a question and the nurse theorist will answer it. For example, Dr. Margaret Newman has a bulletin board that she operates as a part of her Health as Expanding Consciousness Web site. Having the opportunity to ask the theorist a question and receive a response is very exciting.

Dissemination of Information

Nurses who are developing a new theory can use the Internet and the World Wide Web to introduce their theory to the nursing community at large. For a variety of reasons, it is sometimes very difficult to publish a book or have a manuscript published in a peer reviewed journal, and the time lag between the conception of an idea and having it published can be quite lengthy. However, it is relatively simple and quick to publish an article on a Web site. This is both good and bad. It is good for the novice theorist who wishes to have a forum in which to present his or her work, but it is bad in the sense that the work may not be credible, clear, concise, valid, usable, generalizable, or reviewed by others. Just as with anything that is published on the Web, readers must evaluate the credibility of any new theory published online. When reviewing theory on the Web, remember to evaluate the source carefully. On the Web, at least 15 people will think that what you have said is fabulous! (Weinberger, 2002).

When a theorist publishes a theory on the Web, many people read the theory and offer feedback to the theorist. This feedback enables the theorist to make revisions that will hopefully improve the theory. This exposure also creates opportunities for the theorist to locate others who share similar thoughts and interests. Through this exposure, collaborative situations often emerge. One such situation occurred with Dr. Sharon L. Van Sell of the United States and Ioannis A. Kalofissudis of Greece, with their Complexity Nursing Theory. In 2000, Van Sell found Kalofissudis's theory of Holistic Conceptual Development Model of Nursing Science on the Web. Van Sell was very interested in Kalofissudis's theory because conceptually it was very similar to her theory of Nursing Knowledge and Practice. Van Sell traveled to Greece to discuss how they could expand their ideas and make them international in scope. They collaborated and "gave birth" to a new theory called the Complexity Nursing Theory. They are currently completing the final draft of their manuscript for a theory text of the same name (I. Kalofissudis, personal communication sent to Lisa Eichelberger, June 8, 2003). Without the Web, this new theory would most likely have never been developed.

Information technology and the Internet have dramatically changed the way nursing theorists organize, consult, and share information about theory, practice, research, and virtually every aspect of the domain of nursing. The use of information technology and the Internet by the nursing profession will continue to evolve. Such technology holds great potential for nurse theorists to generate, test, and apply knowledge faster and more globally than ever before. It is, however, important to remember that technology is just a tool and the online community is what we make it. It is truly an exciting time to be a nurse theorist, and the best is yet to be.

Learning Activities

1. Imagine how nursing might have been different if Nightingale had had access to the Internet.

2. If Nightingale could have chosen to live in the 1800s or today, which do you think she would choose and why?

3. Review the last 10 postings on the Margaret Newman bulletin board. Summarize the questions, content, and replies.

4. Discuss the types of listservs and discussion groups currently available on the Web for nurses interested in nursing theorists.

5. Formulate one question and post it on a nurse theorist's bulletin board or listserv. Share the responses that you receive with your classmates.

6. Discuss the possible reasons some nurse theorists do not have a presence on the Web. What would it take to create a site for a theorist?

7. Go to the Jones and Bartlett Web site for this text at *http://nursing.jbpub.com* and explore the Web links listed for this chapter.

Feel free to use these blank pages as a canvas for your learning activities.

Lisa Wright Eichelberger— Pioneering Nursing Theory on the World Wide Web

Thinking of oneself as a pioneer is somewhat daunting and oftentimes associated with reaching a certain advanced age. The advanced age part was not something I particularly enjoyed considering. When I was approached about writing a chapter on pioneering nursing theory on the World Wide Web (www), I was somewhat hesitant, not quite seeing the value of such a chapter at first glance. However, after reflection, I agreed. After having authored a nursing theory Web site for almost 15 years, if I have learned nothing else, I have learned two things. The first lesson learned is that few inventions have caused a greater shift in our worldview than that of the Internet, and secondly, the lack of permanency of recorded information on the Web can be a major threat to our knowledge base. We have all experienced the Web phenomena of "here today, gone tomorrow." So it is for those reasons that I have attempted to record a history of nursing theory on the Web and share with you some of my experiences as the webmaster of one of the first nursing theory Web sites. I feel very fortunate to have been a small part in facilitating access to nursing theory knowledge on the Web for those seeking to understand how nursing theory advances the profession of nursing.

The Beginning

I almost left nursing during the 1980s. I was a young nurse, armed with a master's degree, about to embark on doctoral study when I became very disillusioned with what I saw happening in nursing at the national level. You will recall from your study of nursing history that the late 1970s and early 1980s were a rather tumultuous time for the profession primarily because of the American Nurses Association's 1985 proposal looming on the horizon. The 1985 proposal referred to, of course, requiring a baccalaureate degree in nursing for entry into professional practice. While this requirement has yet to become a reality, the proposal caused considerable turmoil and division within the profession for quite some time.

As a nurse educator in my 20s, I served as an associate director of a school of nursing, an opportunity and privilege few have today at such a young age. That leadership position afforded me the foray into the national arena, where I quickly became disillusioned and discouraged with the nursing profession. I witnessed grown women yelling and screaming at one another during national educational meetings and using irrational and illogical arguments while debating entry into practice. This type of defeatist behavior and lack of vision on the part of nursing made me seriously consider leaving the profession. I was not sure that I wanted to continue to be a part of a profession that was so divided and whose leaders demonstrated such unreasonable and unprofessional behavior.

But during that time, I also had the good fortune to discover something else about nursing—the beauty and wisdom of nursing theory. I can honestly say that if it had not been for the study of nursing theory, I might not have remained in nursing. The disillusionment and discouragement that I was feeling in my professional life was overcome by the excitement and pure joy I found in studying the work of nurse theorists. I remained in nursing because of the intellectual challenge I encountered when analyzing nursing theory.

During my doctoral study at the University of Alabama at Birmingham, I discovered a completely new and different way of thinking when studying the work of nursing theorists. Martha Rogers's work was particularly intriguing and thought provoking for me. I remember thinking after reading Rogers's "*Little*

Purple Book (1970) and the *Tao of Physics* (Capra, 1975) how much nursing had to offer that was intellectually stimulating and thought provoking. And while there was a certain amount of craziness being demonstrated almost on a daily basis around me, I found a place where I could focus my thoughts and hopes.

My worldview changed after reading Rogers's *Science of Unitary Man*. Rogers's theory, in particular, made me question everything about the way I viewed nursing and my worldview. It helped me to understand the complexities of the science that is nursing, and I rediscovered what I had originally loved about nursing. Rogers's *Science of Unitary Human Man* did that for me. While studying at University of Alabama at Birmingham, I was afforded the opportunity to personally meet and study with many of the early nurse theorists, and I was so inspired by them and their true pioneering thinking; it made me proud to be a nurse.

So I became a lover of theory, embracing it, using it, and relying on it to frame my approach to patient care. I turned inward, if you will, from focusing on the disorganization that was occurring at the national level of nursing and focused rather on my views of nursing and how nursing theory could change one's entire approach to nursing practice and research. Nursing theory saved nursing for me, and I think it is for that reason that I have devoted so much of my personal time to advancing nursing theory on the Web.

The Web

Those of us who became nurses in the 1970s have experienced two revolutionary events in our careers—the development of AIDS and the development of the Internet. We can all remember starting IVs and attending deliveries without wearing gloves and spending hours in the basements of libraries gathering information and learning without the help of the Internet. I think most would agree that both occurrences have radically changed nursing.

Humans have always had the need to communicate with others, and so it is not hard to understand the success of the Web. The Web is simply a worldwide system of interconnected networks and computers that allows us to communicate with one another in a very fast and immediate way that is not limited by proximity. But I think few in 1970 could have imagined our dependence on it today.

While the exact timing, purpose, and development of what is known as the Web and the Internet can be debated, I think most would agree that the desire for resource sharing that occurred in the early 1970s was at the heart of this development. It was not until the mid-1980s that the Web began being used for daily computer communications and electronic mail (e-mail) began being used broadly across communities to provide electronic communication between people.

Nursing Theory on the Web

If you study the evolution of the World Wide Web, it is easy to see the parallels with nursing theory. The development of the Web mirrors the development of nursing theory as a whole with the foundations of both being laid in the 1800s and the early 1900s, much work being accomplished in the 1960s-1970s, and huge advances being made in the 1980s and 90s.

The existence of nursing theory on the Internet began in the 1990s, but it is unclear which nurse theorist Web site was actually the first to be activated. Unfortunately, most of those who created nursing theory Web sites did not record publicly on their sites when the site was first posted. Unlike a publication date that records the point in time any new book is written, many, if not most, of the theory Web sites have no traceable histories.

There are some nurse theorists who currently have no Web presence. In 1996, when I first started working with nursing theory on the Web, I created a list of major nursing theorists without any Web sites and extended a standing offer to work with anyone who had the desire to create Web sites for these theorists. Unfortunately, the list of nursing theorists without Web sites has changed very little since 1996.

It was my desire that every nurse theorist have a Web presence, so I created a site for Dr. Ernestine Wiedenbach in 1996 that can be found at http://

nursing.clayton.edu/eichelberger/wiedenbach.htm. I chose to create a site for Wiedenbach because she was a maternal/infant nurse like me and not because I personally used Wiedenbach's theory. It is still my hope that one day every nurse theorist will have a Web site to increase available information for nurses—even those without ready access to libraries and theory texts. I think many of us, particularly those of us who live in the United States, can't imagine not having access to information with our extensive library system and interlibrary loans, etc. But for many people, particularly those not currently enrolled in an educational program, the availability of information and textbooks can be limited. Access to the Internet is much more widespread than libraries, underlining the importance of publishing information about theorists on the Internet.

Compilation Web Sites

The history of two nursing theory compilation or repository sites is known. Compilation or repository nursing theory Web sites are those that list links to existing nursing theory sites rather than providing direct theoretical information. Both compilation sites were established in 1996 and have remained in operation since that time. The first site is the Nursing Theory Page (NTP), at http://www.sandiego.edu/academics/nursing/theory/, which began in early 1996. In the fall of 1996, the Clayton State University (CSU) nursing theory Web site was launched at http://nursing.clayton.edu/eichelberger/nursing.htm. I published that site and have maintained its content and links since its inception.

Both sites were created as a community service for the purpose of advancing the study and use of nursing theory through increasing access to nursing theory knowledge and facilitating connections between nurses interested in using theory in their practice. This service was provided at no cost to the seeker at a time when finding information about nursing theory on the Web was much more difficult that it is today. It is important to remember that in 1996, when the CSU theory site was first started, browsing the Internet was much more difficult than it is today. Search engines were much more limited, the now-ubiquitous Google did not even exist, and most webmasters did not understand the ways in which one could lead seekers to a site. A search one day may yield entirely different results than one conducted the next day using the same search parameters.

The NTP, which began on May 21, 1996, provides links to multiple nursing theory Web sites, as well as information about theory conferences and other related sources (Donnelly, 2001). This Web site is the collaborative effort of a now-defunct international nursing theory group and is currently supported by the University of San Diego. Judy Norris at the University of Alberta served as the first Webmaster for the site until the site was transferred to the servers at the University of San Diego and Ann M. Mayo, RN, DNSc, took over the maintenance of the site.

The CSU theory compilation Web site began as a project of undergraduate students in my nursing theory class in the fall of 1996. Understanding the value of facilitating the search for information about nursing theory started by my students, I revamped and expanded the CSU site and have served as the webmaster since the fall of 1996. Clayton State University has provided the server space and support for the site since its beginning. Other compilation sites have come and gone during the past 13 years, but these two sites have consistently provided information about nursing theory on the Web and responded to seekers of information about nursing theory.

Managing the CSU Theory Web Site

Once the theory Web site was uploaded, I began to receive e-mails from nursing students all over the world right away. All were seeking help in locating resources about the various nurse theorists. It was so exciting to check my inbox and to find inquiries from students, especially those in foreign countries. When I was not able to locate a resource for the student, I always asked that when and if they located information on the Web that they thought would be helpful to others, that they share it with me so that I could make it available for others on the Web site.

In addition to e-mails from theory students, shortly after publishing the CSU compilation site, I received a rather disconcerting e-mail from one of the members of the international nursing theory group demanding that I immediately take down the Web site. This individual was very unhappy that another site had been created that led others to theory Web sites. I was taken aback to say the least and for a period of time found myself in a rather heated debate with members of the NTP community.

After a period of time and much discussion, we were able to develop a better understanding of the work and purposes of both sites and an appreciation of the contributions that all were making in advancing nursing theory. Judy Norris, in particular, was most gracious in acknowledging and helping others realize that no one owned the Internet. And so the two sites agreed to cross-list each other's site, to share information, and work together. Several years later, at a Rogerian conference, I had the opportunity to meet the person who wrote the original e-mail telling me to take down my Web site. We never spoke of the incident.

Lessons Learned

Serving as "web diva" for the CSU site has been a rare opportunity, and it has been a labor of love. The most gratifying aspect of managing the theory Web site has to have been the privilege of communicating directly with the nurse theorists themselves via e-mail, and corresponding with nurses from all over the world who are interested in theory.

Managing the Web site has gotten easier over time. The volume of e-mail has lessened as students have become more savvy in searching for information, as sites have become more stable, and as more and more search engines have made searching easier.

I have learned that nursing theorists are, for the most part, very generous people who delight in sharing their knowledge and expertise with others. With the advent of e-mail, seekers have the opportunity to communicate directly with experts in various nursing theories. Some theorists themselves participate in online discussions with seekers. Kathy Kolcaba, Margaret Newman, Savina Schoenhofer, and Imogene King were a few who frequently communicated with students and others about their theories. In 2007, Dr. Imogene King passed away at the age of 84, but until shortly before her death, she routinely answered students' e-mails.

Lack of permanency of information on the Web remains an area of concern. Because information can be posted one day and removed the next, access to a sizable amount of information is lost over time. I have tried to capture information that I thought was particularly useful and needed to be preserved. I always obtain permission from the original author of the site prior to reposting the information. When this happens I create a new site within my nursing theory Web site so that the information can be maintained for others. One example is the memorial for Virginia Henderson that was originally published on the Sigma Theta Tau Web site until 1999 when it was removed. Believing that all future students of theory should have access to this information, I obtained permission from Sigma Theta Tau to permanently display the tribute at http://nursing.clayton.edu/eichelberger/in_celebration_of_virginia_avene. htm. Another example is a paper discussing Johnson's behavioral systems theory. It was removed in 2002 and then reposted on my Web site at http:// nursing.clayton.edu/eichelberger/theory/johnson_behavioral_system.htm.

One of the areas where I see a real need and potential to advance the understanding of nursing theory is that of discussion based electronic mailing lists or list servs. List servs are automatic mailing list servers that individuals join with their e-mail addresses. When an e-mail is addressed to a LISTSERV mailing list, it is automatically broadcast to everyone on the list. The result is similar to a newsgroup or forum, except that the messages are transmitted as e-mail and are therefore available only to individuals on the list. Participants routinely post questions in the form of an e-mail blast to the entire list serv membership and anyone can offer an answer or opinion. List servs are somewhat time consuming to maintain, and it is for that reason, I suspect, that many of the theorist groups have abandoned the support for them. Parse's group remains the most active electronic mailing list.

Great insights exist in the list serv postings—particularly if the actual theorists and experts who personally worked with the theorists agree to participate. Many of the original theorists are retiring, and many have passed away; the discussions that have occurred on some of the electronic mailing lists contained very valuable explanations and applications, but are often lost when the electronic mailing lists are discontinued.

For the first 5 years or so, I did not record the number of hits the site received. Since I began recording, the site has received almost 700,000 hits. In the first 7 years or so, I never received solicitations to advertise on my site; however, the past 4 or so years have seen a rise in requests for advertisement and requests for me to add sites that were not directly related to theory for commercial reasons. No advertisements have ever been a part of the CSU site. I am very gratified, however, when nurse theorists contact me directly and ask that I add their site to my Web site, or authors contact me and ask that I list their book or their videos about nursing theory on the site.

One of the most fortuitous hits on my site was that of Dr. Kathleen Sitzman, my coauthor in writing *Understanding the Work of the Nurse Theorist: A Creative Beginning*. Dr. Sitzman and I have never met in person, and yet in 2003, we began a virtual partnership that led to the publishing of our text. I received a phone call one day from someone introducing herself as a lover of nursing theory and asking if I would be interested in collaborating with her on a nursing theory textbook. Because of my Web site, she thought that she would like to work with me. Thus began our long-distance collaboration.

I appreciate having the opportunity to share with you my experiences in serving as webmaster for a nursing theory Web site. I must say I am very grateful for the class assignment that started it all many years ago. I have long since lost touch with the two students who gave birth to the Web site, but I want to thank them for giving me the idea that led to one of the most rewarding creative outlets I have had in nursing. It has been a lovely journey.

Glossary

aesthetics (nursing art) The perception of deep meanings within nursing practice that evoke creativity and result in multilevel understandings and expressions of practice within an artistic context.

assumption Principles that are accepted as being true without proof or concrete verification, usually based on logic, inductive reasoning, or deductive reasoning.

concept An abstraction (thought, model, mental formation) based on the observation of phenomena.

deductive reasoning Formation of specific predictions based on general observations or principles.

domain A territory or field of activity. In nursing practice, generally four domains are recognized: empirics (scientific competence), personal (therapeutic use of self), ethics (moral/ethical comportment), and aesthetics (transformative art/acts).

empirics Replicating, validating, explaining, and structuring. Expressed as knowledge by theories and models and integrated into practice as scientific competence.

ethics A system of moral values that is concerned with "doing the right thing" that is associated with trust, respect, dignity, human/legal rights of the nurse and client and is based on the consensus of the population involved in the transaction.

grand theory A theory that represents the broad concepts within an entire discipline (e.g., nursing).

hypothesis A statement of a relationship between variables that can be tested.

idea A mental conception or image.

inductive reasoning Formation of general predictions based on specific observations.

knowledge Perception of reality developed through insight, learning, and investigation expressed in a form that can be shared. It is collectively assessed as valuable through shared understanding.

medical model   The approach to the diagnosis and treatment of illness as practiced by physicians in the West. The physician focuses on the patient's defect or dysfunction. The medical history, physical examination, and diagnostic tests provide the basis for the identification and treatment of a specific illness or condition.

metaparadigm   Refers to an overall worldview (e.g., reductionism, rationalism, relativism, etc.). See also *paradigm*.

middle-range theory (practice theory)   A theory that focuses on one part of a discipline in an attempt to explain and predict phenomena. Such theories are meant to be directly applicable to everyday nursing practice.

moral/ethical comportment   Expression of ethical knowledge and knowing in nursing practice.

nondualism   The assertion that everything in the universe is unavoidably interconnected and can never be completely separated into distinct parts. The belief that everything affects everything else to varying degrees.

nursing model   A symbolic rendering of ideas or concepts with pictorial elements that illustrates the relationships between and among the ideas or concepts.

nursing process   A structured organizational framework for nursing that includes: assessment, nursing diagnosis, planning, implementation, and evaluation.

nursing science   The systematic exploration, measurement, and explanation of phenomena specific to nursing. Also refers to the body of knowledge that is specific to nursing.

paradigm   The lens through which the world is viewed by an individual, group, or discipline. A way of assigning value or worth to observations, knowledge, methods, and phenomena. See also *metaparadigm*.

phenomenon   Any event that can be sensed, attended to, or apprehended by a sentient being.

philosophy   A system of beliefs about the general nature of things, particularly morality, ethics, and how the world should be viewed. The study of principles underlying human thought, conduct, and understandings about the nature of where we fit in the universe.

postmodern nursing   A movement toward knowledge discovery that does not rely exclusively on empirical evidence of phenomena but that also focuses on the discovery of the meaning of phenomena. This is a sort of "learn as you go" approach that is done by immersing oneself in a phenomena of interest, trying to discern pattern and meaning, while acknowledging the unavoidable interconnectedness of the observer (self) with the phenomenon. See also *empirics*.

research   Planned, deliberate study of a specific phenomenon for the purpose of deepening understanding and allowing for prediction and replication of the phenomenon.

scientific medicine   Care focused on the illness, not the client. The process of diagnosis depends on structured knowledge that is accepted by the mainstream medical community. Medications, surgeries, and traditional treatments are the focus of practice.

theoretical physics   Speculative study and conjecture regarding the interactions, properties, and changes associated with matter and energy.

theory   An abstract generalization that presents a systematic explanation about the relationships among phenomena. A nursing theory is a theory that is meant to address phenomena specific to nursing practice.

therapeutic use of self   Expression of a personal knowledge and knowing in nursing practice that is integrated with ethics, empiric knowledge, and nursing art.

wholism   Being aware of the interaction of many parts, or aspects, that form a whole system.

References

Alligood, M. R. (Interviewer). (n.d.). *The nurse theorists: Portrait of excellence* (Vol. 2). [Online interview of Pat Benner]. Helene Fuld Foundation FITNE. Available from *http://www.fitne.net/vlrc4/nurse_theorists1.jsp;jsessionid=89CF957ABC233E27A7AA0A653E803807*

Alligood, M. R., Krivicich, D., Kramer, A. S., Erickson, H. C., & Mishel, M. H. (2008). *The nurse theorists portraits of excellence* (Vol. 2). [Video recording]. Athens, OH: FITNE.

Allmark, P. (2003). Popper and Nursing Theory. *Nursing Philosophy, 4* (1), 13–16.

Ayers, A. (1990). *Language, truth, and logic* (2nd ed.) London: Penguin.

Barrett, E. A. M. (1990). *Visions of Rogers' science-based nursing.* New York: National League for Nursing Press.

Benner, P. (1984). *From novice to expert: Excellence and power in clinical nursing practice.* Menlo Park, CA: Addison-Wesley.

Benner, P., Hooper-Kyriakidis, P., & Stannard, D. (1999). *Clinical wisdom in critical care: A thinking-in-action approach.* Philadelphia, PA: W. B. Saunders.

Benner, P., & Wrubel, J. (1989). *The primacy of caring: Stress and coping in health and illness.* Menlo Park, CA: Addison-Wesley.

Biley, F. C. (2002). *Theory: An overview of the Science of Unitary Human Beings.* Posted on the Unitary Health Care Web page in 2002, written in the early 1990s. Retrieved May 30, 2003, from: *http://medweb.uwcm.ac.uk/martha/theory.htm*

Brykczynski, L. A. (1999). An interpretive study describing the clinical judgment of nursing practitioners. *Scholarly Inquiry for Nursing Practice: An International Journal, 13*(2), 141–166.

Capra, F. (1975). *The tao of physics.* Retrieved January 29, 2010, from http://users.telenet.be/sterf/texts/science/The_Tao_of_Physics.pdf

Cash, K. (2001). Theory as resistance. *Nursing Philosophy, 2,* 1–3.

Chinn, P. L., & Kramer, M. K. (1999). *Theory and nursing: Integrated knowledge development.* St. Louis, MO: Mosby.

Cowling, W. R. (1990). A template for nursing practice. In E. A. M. Barret (Ed.), *Visions of Rogers' science-based nursing* (pp. 45–65). New York: National League for Nursing Press.

Crotty, M. (1998). *Foundations of social research: Meaning and perspective in the research process.* London: Sage.

Deering, C. G., & Eichelberger, L. W. (2002). Mirror mirror on the wall: Using online discussion groups to improve interpersonal skills. CIN: *Computer, Informatics, Nursing, 20,* 150–156.

Dickoff, J., & James, P. (1968). A theory of theories: A position paper. *Nursing Research, 17,* 197–203.

Donnelly, E. (2001). An assessment of nursing theories as guides to scientific inquiry. In N. L. Chaska (Ed.), *The nursing profession tomorrow and beyond* (p. 332). Thousand Oaks, CA: Sage.

Drevdahl, D. (1999). Sailing beyond: Nursing theory and the person. *Advances in Nursing Science, 21*(4), 1–13.

Dreyfus, S. E., & Dreyfus, H. I. (1980). *A five-stage model of the mental activities involved in directed skill acquisition.* Unpublished report. Berkeley: University of California at Berkeley.

Eichelberger, L. W. (1991). Retrieved May 28, 2003, from "In Celebration of Virginia," *http://www.healthsci.clayton.edu/eichelberger/in_celebration_of_Virginia_avene.htm*

Evers, G. C. M. (2001). Naming nursing: Evidence-based nursing. *Nursing Diagnosis, 12*(4), 137–141.

Fawcett, J. (2000). *Analysis and evaluation of contemporary nursing knowledge: Nursing models and theories.* Philadelphia: Davis.

Fawcett, J. (2005). *Contemporary nursing knowledge: Analysis and evaluation of nursing models and theories* (2nd ed.). Philadelphia: Davis.

Fuld, H. *Nurse Theorists: Portraits of Excellence.* prod. FITNE, Inc., Athens, Ohio, 1987–89, video series.

George, J. B. (2002). *Nursing theories: The base for professional nursing practice.* Upper Saddle River, NJ: Prentice Hall.

Glazer, S. (2000). *Postmodern nursing.* Retrieved May 30, 2003, from *http://www.thepublicinterest.com/archives/2000summer/article1.html*

Henderson, V. ([1960] 1997). *Basic principles of nursing care.* Washington, DC: American Nurses Publishing.

Hubble Space Telescope Web site. (2003). Retrieved May 28, 2003, from *http://www.stsci.edu/hst/HST_overview/*

Ingram, R. (1991). Why does nursing need theory? *Journal of Advanced Nursing, 16,* 350–353.

Johns, C. (1995). Framing learning through reflection within Carper's fundamental ways of knowing in nursing. *Journal of Advanced Nursing, 22*(2), 226–234.

Johns, C. C. (1993). Guided reflection. In A. Palmer, S. Burns, & C. Bulman (Eds.), *Reflective practice in nursing: Growth of the professional practitioner* (pp. 110–130). Oxford: Blackwell Scientific.

Kalisch, P. A., & Kalisch, B. J. (1995). *The advance of American nursing* (3rd ed.). Philadelphia: Lippincott Williams & Wilkins.

King, I. M. (1971). *Toward a theory for nursing: General concepts of human behavior.* New York, NY: John Wiley and Sons.

King, I. M. (1981). A theory for nursing: Systems, concept, process. New York, NY: John Wiley and Sons.

King, I. M. (1986). Curriculum and instruction in nursing. Norwalk, CT: Appleton-Century-Crofts.

King, I. M. (1990). Health as the goal for nursing. *Nursing Science Quarterly, 3,* 123–128.

King, I. M. (1996). The theory of goal attainment in research and practice. *Nursing Science Quarterly, 2,* 61–66.

King, I. M. (1997). King's theory of goal attainment in practice. *Nursing Science Quarterly, 10,* 180–185.

King, I. M. (2006). Imogene M. King's theory of goal attainment. In M. E. Parker (Ed.), *Nursing theorist & nursing practice* (2nd ed., pp. 235–267). Philadelphia: Davis.

King, I. M. (2007). King's structure, process, and outcome in the 21st century. In C. L. Sieloff & M. A. Frey (Eds.). *Middle range theory development: Using King's conceptual system,* New York, NY: Springer Publishing.

Kolcaba, K. (1994). A theory of holistic comfort for nursing. *Journal of Advanced Nursing, 19,* 1178–1184.

Kolcaba, K. (1996). A holistic perspective on comfort care as an advance directive. *Critical Care Nursing Quarterly, 18*(4), 66–79.

Kolcaba, K. (2003). Comfort theory and practice: A vision for holistic health care and research. New York: Springer-Verlag.

Lazarus, R. S. (1966). *Psychological stress and the coping process.* New York, NY: McGraw-Hill.

Leininger, M. (1978). *Transcultural nursing: Concepts, theories, and practices.* New York, NY: John Wiley and Sons.

Leininger, M. (1981). *Care: An essential human need.* Detroit, MI: Wayne State University Press.

Leininger, M. (1991). *Culture care diversity and universality: A theory of nursing.* New York, NY: National League for Nursing Press.

Leininger, M. (1995). *Transcultural nursing: Concepts, theories, and practices* (2nd ed.). Blacklic, OH: McGraw Hill and Greyden Press.

Leininger, M. (2001). *Culture care diversity and universality: A theory of nursing.* Sudbury, MA: Jones and Bartlett Publishers.

Leininger, M. (2002). *Transcultural nursing: Concepts, theories, research, and practices* (3rd ed.). Blacklic, OH: McGraw Hill Professional.

Levine, M. E. (1989). The conservation principles of nursing: Twenty years later. In M. E. Riehl-Sisca (Ed.), *Conceptual models for nursing practice* (3rd ed., pp. 325–337). Norwalk, CT: Appleton & Lange.

Marchione, J. (1993). *Margaret Newman: Health as Expanding Consciousness.* Newbury Park, CA: Sage.

Messmer, P. R. (2009). *Portrait in professionalism: Imogene M. King.* Retrieved January 29, 2010, from http://www.nursinglibrary.org/Portal/main.aspx?pageid=4024&sid =9863

Montgomery, B. (2000). *Florence Nightingale: Mystic, visionary, reformer.* Springhouse, PA: Springhouse Publishing.

Mosby's Medical, Nursing, & Allied Health Dictionary (5th ed.). (1998). St. Louis, MO: Mosby.

Neuman, B., & Fawcett, J. (2002). *The Neuman Systems Model* (4th ed.). Upper Saddle River, NJ: Prentice Hall.

Newman, M. (2000). *Health as expanding consciousness* (2nd ed.). Sudbury, MA: Jones and Bartlett Publishing, National League for Nursing.

Newman, M. (2003). "Overview of the Theory." Retrieved May 30, 2003, from *http://www.healthasexpandingconsciousness.org*

Nightingale, F. (1859). *Notes on nursing: What it is, and what it is not.* Philadelphia: Edward Stern and Company.

Orem, D. E. (2001). *Nursing: Concepts and practice* (6th ed.). St. Louis, MO: Mosby.

Orlando, I. J. (1990). *The dynamic nurse–patient relationship: Function, process, and principles.* New York: National League for Nursing. (Reprinted from 1961, New York: G.P. Putnam's Sons.)

Orlando, I. J. (1972). *The Discipline and teaching of nursing process*. New York: G.P. Putnam's Sons.

Parse, R.R. (1981). *Man-living-health*: A *theory of nursing*. New York, NY: John Wiley and Sons.

Parse, R. R. (1987). *Nursing science: Major paradigms, theories, and critiques*. Philadelphia, PA: W. B. Saunders.

Parse, R. R. (1989). Essentials for practicing the art of nursing. *Nursing Science Quarterly*, *2*, 111.

Parse, R. R. (1990). Health: A personal commitment. *Nursing Science Quarterly*, *3*, 136–140.

Parse, R. R. (1992). Human becoming: Parse's theory of nursing. *Nursing Science Quarterly*, *5*, 35–42.

Parse, R. R. (1995). *Illuminations: The human becoming theory in practice and research*. New York, NY: National League for Nursing.

Parse, R. R. (1996). The human becoming: Challenges in practice and research. *Nursing Science Quarterly*, *9*, 55–60.

Parse, R. R. (1998). *The human becoming school of thought: A perspective for nurses and other health professionals*. Thousand Oaks, CA: Sage.

Peden, A. R. (1998). The evolution of an intervention—the use of Peplau's process of practice-based theory development. *Journal of Psychiatric and Mental Health Nursing, 5*, 173–178.

Pender, N. J. (1996). *Health promotion in nursing practice* (3rd ed.). Stamford, CT: Appleton & Lange.

Pender, N. J. (2003). Information retrieved May 27, 2003, from *http://www.nursing. umich.edu/faculty/pender/pender_questions.html*

Pender, N. J., Murdaugh, C. L., & Parsons, M. A. (2002). *Health promotion in nursing practice* (4th ed.). Upper Saddle River, NJ: Prentice Hall.

Peplau, H. E. (1952). *Interpersonal relations in nursing*. New York: G. P. Putnam's Sons.

Peplau, H. E. (1988). *Interpersonal relations in nursing*. London: The Macmillan Press Limited.

Peplau, H. E. (1989). Theory: The professional dimension. In A. O. O'Toole & S. Welt (Eds.), *Interpersonal theory in nursing practice: Selected works of Hildegard E. Peplau* (pp. 21–30). New York: Springer.

Peplau, H. E. (1997). Peplau's theory of interpersonal relations. *Nursing Science Quarterly, 10*(4), 162–167.

Reed, P. G., & Shearer, N. B. C. (2009) *Perspectives on nursing theory* (5th ed.). Philadelphia, PA: Lippincott Williams & Wilkins.

Reed, P. G., Shearer, N. B. C., & Nicoll, L. H. (2004). *Perspectives on nursing theory* (4th ed.). Philadelphia, PA: Lippincott Williams & Wilkins.

Rogers, M. E. (1970). *An introduction to the theoretical basis of nursing*. Philadelphia: Davis.

Rogers, M. E. (1992). Nursing science and the space age. *Nursing Science Quarterly, 5*, 27–34.

Rogers, M. E. (1994). Educating the nurse for the future. In V. M. Malinski & E. A. M. Barrett (Eds.), *Martha Rogers: Her life and work* (pp. 61–68). Philadelphia: Davis.

Roy, C. (1970). Adaptation: A conceptual framework for nursing. *Nursing Outlook, 18*(3), 42–45.

Roy, C. (1984). *Introduction to nursing: An adaptation model* (2nd ed.). Upper Saddle River, NJ: Prentice Hall.

Roy, C., & Andrews, H. A. (1999). *The Roy Adaptation Model* (2nd ed.). Stamford, CT: Appleton & Lange.

Samten, Losang. (1999). Mandala. Philadelphia Museum of Art. Retrieved May 21, 2003, from *http://www.philadelphiamuseum.org*

Schiller, D. (1994). *The Little Zen Companion.* New York: Workman Publishing.

Seurat. G. (1884–1886). *A Sunday on La Grand Jatte* [Oil on canvas, 208 x 308 cm]. Chicago: The Art Institute of Chicago.

Seurat, G. (1884–1886). *Bathers at Asnieres* [Oil painting, 201 x 300 cm]. London: National Gallery.

Tomey, A. M., & Alligood, M. R. (2002). *Nursing theorists and their work* (5th ed.). St. Louis, MO: Mosby.

Tomey, A. M., & Alligood, M. R. (2006). *Nursing theorists and their work* (6th ed.). St. Louis, MO: Mosby.

Van Sell, S. L., & Kalofissudis, I. A. (2003). Formulating nursing theory. Retrieved June 4, 2003 from *http://www.nursing.gr/theory/theory.html*

Watson, J. (1988). New dimensions of human caring theory. *Nursing Science Quarterly, 1*(4), 175–181.

Watson, J. (1999, Summer issue). Aesthetic expressions of caring: Private psalms—surrendering to the sacred. Personal professional reflections on caring and healing. *International Journal of Human Caring, 3*(1).

Watson, J. (2003). Information retrieved May 1, 2003, from *http://www.uchsc.edu/nursing/caring*

Watson, J. (2005). *Caring science as sacred science.* Philadelphia: Davis.

Weinberger, D. (2002). *Small pieces loosely joined: A unified theory of the Web.* Cambridge, MA: Perseus Publishing.

Wiedenbach, E. (2003). Guide to Ernestine Wiedenbach papers, Yale University. Information retrieved May 28, 2003, from *http://webtext.library.yale.edu/xml2html /mssa.1647.con.html#top*

Wilde, M. H. (1999). Why embodiment now? *Advances in Nursing Science, 22*(2), 25–38.

Suggested Readings

Meleis, A. (1985). *Theoretical nursing: Development and progress.* Philadelphia: Lippincott.

Polit, D. F., & Hungler, B. P. (1999). *Nursing research: Principles and methods* (6th ed.), Philadelphia: Lippincott Williams & Wilkins.

Index

Color Plate 5.1   Example of pointillism.

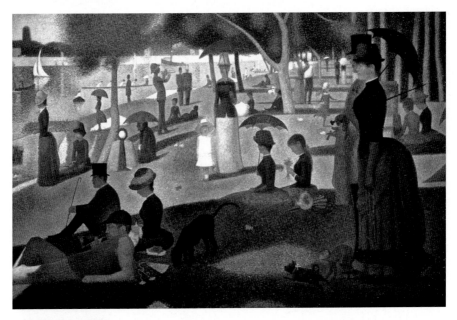

Color Plate 5.2   Seurat, Georges, French, 1859–1891, **A Sunday on La Grande Jatte—1884**, 1884–1886, oil on canvas, 207.6 x 308 cm, Helen Birch Bartlett Memorial Collection, 1926. 224.
Reprinted with permission from The Art Institute of Chicago.

Color Plate 10.1 A mandala. This and other mandalas can be found at *http://www.mandali.com*.
Mandala was created by Cyl and is used with permission.

Color Plate 10.2 Floor of Amiens Cathedral, Amiens, France.
Photo taken by Robert Ferre. Used with permission.

Color Plate 10.3 People walking the floor of Amiens Cathedral, Amiens, France.
Photo taken by Robert Ferre. Used with permission.

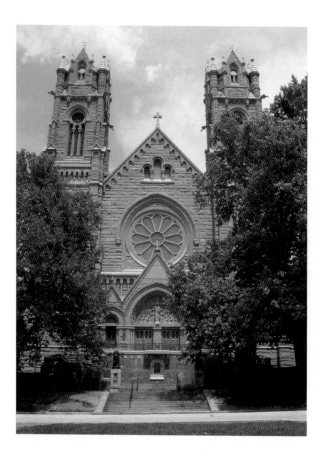

Color Plate 10.4
The Cathedral of the Madeline in Salt Lake City, Utah.
Photo taken by Rick Sitzman. Used with permission.

Color Plate 10.5 Baptismal font inside the Cathedral of the Madeline in Salt Lake City, Utah.

Photo taken by Rick Sitzman. Used with permission.

Color Plate 10.6 This Sand Mandala was created in June 2003 at the Philadelphia Museum of Art by Venerable Losang Samten. It represents the cycle of life and death.

Color Plate 10.7 Kincardine Labyrinth Peace Garden, Geddes Environmental Park in Kincardine, Ontario, Canada.

Photo taken by Donald and Glynda Matheson. Used with permission.

Color Plate 11.1

Student illustration
Myra Estrine Levine Mandala.

Conservation: Symbolized by a light bulb in the center. Light bulbs give light and are productive. Light bulbs also symbolize ideas… theories are ideas.

Historicity: Genetics. The hearts show dominant (dark pink) and recessive (light pink) traits.

Specificity: Different pathways are coming from the center of the light bulb representing the multiple stimulus response pathways.

Redundancy: If one pathway can't get the job done, another pathway will compensate.

Amy Davis Arreaza, MSN, FNP-BC.

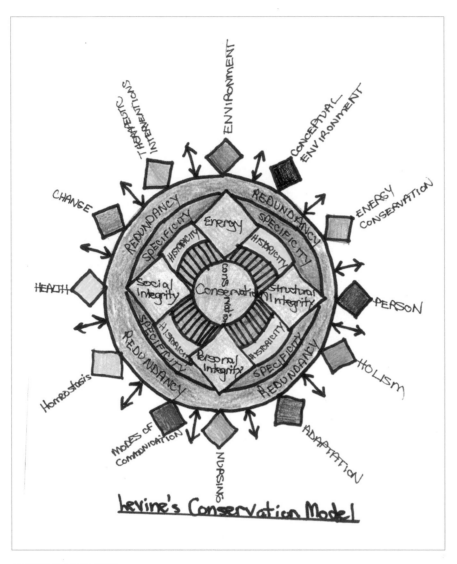

Color Plate 11.2 Student illustration **Levine's Conservation Model**.
Nancy Capponi, RN, BSN, Masters Student, Clayton State University.

Student illustration
**Betty Neuman's Theory
Interpreted Through
Mandala Art**.
The large circle in
the center is the focal
point and includes the
symbol for Maslow's
hierarchy of needs:
physiological, sociocultural,
developmental, spiritual.
The concentric circles
around the center signify
client (brown triangle
with a circle on top),
environment (blue clouds
and yellow circle sunshine),
health (red crosses), and
nursing (pink hearts).
Amy Davis Arreaza, MSN, FNP-BC.

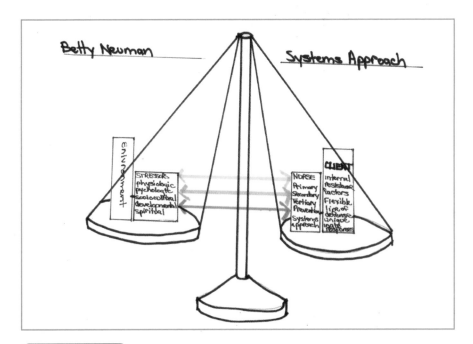

Student illustration **Betty Neuman's System Approach**.
Nancy Capponi, RN, BSN, Masters Student, Clayton State University.

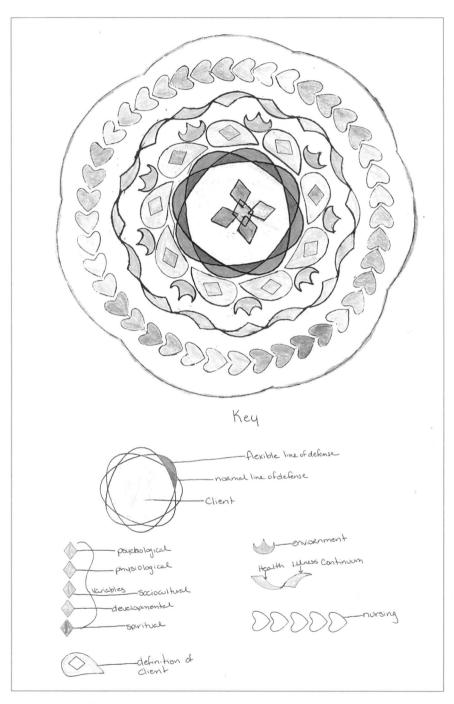

Key

flexible line of defense
normal line of defense
Client

psychological
physiological
Variables — sociocultural
developmental
spiritual

enviornment
Health illness Continuum

nursing

definition of
client

Student illustration **Betty Neuman's System Model Mandala**.
Rita Colella, RN, MSN, APN

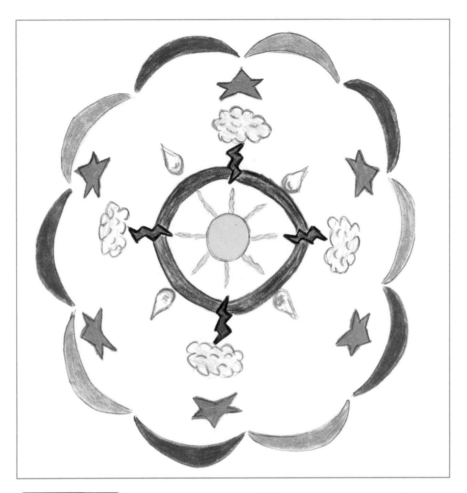

Color Plate 13.1 Student illustration **Mandala Representing Roy's Adaptation Model**.

This mandala representing Roy's Adaptation Model was created to show the grouping of related/connected units that form a unified whole (environment/ nature) and the adaptations that human beings undertake while living within an unpredictable natural environment. The "client/client system" is the central or focal point and is represented by the sun, the four modes of adaptation are represented by the four lightning bolts (representative of activity/energy and interaction needed to adapt), the four major concepts are represented by the clouds, the stars represent the nursing process, and the crescent moons represent the ten supporting scientific and philosophical concepts.

This mandala utilizes symbols from nature to conceptualize Roy's theory that focuses on human beings as an adaptive system, and as such must also adapt to the environment and the forces of nature. It reveals our continual interaction with environmental stimuli.

Noreen Frodella, BSN, RN, BC, graduate student, William Paterson University.

Color Plate 13.2 Student illustration **Interpretation of Roy's Model Through Mandala Art**.

Models of adaptation:

The light blue interior heart symbolizes the physiologic.

The pink heart surrounding the interior blue heart symbolizes self concept.

The smaller hearts scattered around the center represent role function and knowing self amidst others.

The arrows signify interdependence, giving, and receiving.

The four major concepts are located in the center pink heart: client is the human figure, environment is represented by the mug of coffee he is holding (stimulus), health is represented by the cross behind the human figure, and nursing is symbolized by the yellow shoes (support given to promote adaptation).

Nursing process is represented by the encircling stethoscope.

Philosophical concept is represented by the star because human meaning is rooted in the universe.

Amy Davis Arreaza, MSN, FNP-BC.

Color Plate 14.1   Student illustration **Interpretation of Orem's Theory Through Mandala Art**.

Self care: The flag design represents independence. People are independent when they do what they can to maintain life, health, and well-being.

Self-care deficit: The handicap symbol, made into a compass, symbolizes dependency of the patient coupled with the guidance, direction, and support of the nurse.

Nursing systems: Represented by the fish and hook because it reminds me of the saying: "Give a man a fish, feed him for a day. Teach a man to fish, feed him for a lifetime." The nurse compensates for what the patient cannot do for himself while teaching how to care for himself.

Nursing process: All the symbols are encompassed in a larger symbol—an apothecary symbol. This symbol represents diagnosis and prescription, determining why nursing care is needed.

Amy Davis Arreaza, MSN, FNP-BC.

Color Plate 15.1

Student illustration **Leininger Mandala**. We really are a global community. Our cultures overlap and are interwoven. The shapes are identical and not one is better or more important than the other. The hearts represent caring, which is non-cultural specific. Caring is universal.

Amy Davis Arreaza, MSN, FNP-BC.

Color Plate 16.1 Origami bird. Created by Aaron Sitzman.

Color Plate 16.2 Origami shapes. Created by Aaron Sitzman.

Color Plate 23.1 Star Cluster Hodge 301 in the Tarantula Nebula. Photo taken in 1999 by the Hubble Space Telescope.

Color Plate 23.2 30 Doradus Nebula. Photo taken in 2001 by the Hubble Space Telescope.